An Introduction to Ethics for Nurses

An Introduction to Ethics for Nurses

Richard H Rowson
Principal Lecturer in Philosophy,
Polytechnic of Wales

Scutari Press

© Scutari Press 1990

A division of Scutari Projects, the publishing company of the Royal College of Nursing

First published 1990

British Library Cataloguing in Publication Data
Rowson, Richard
    An introduction to ethics for nurses.
    1. Medicine. Nursing. Ethical aspects
    I. Title
    174.2

    ISBN 1-871364-40-X

Typeset by MC Typeset Ltd., Gillingham
Printed and bound in Great Britain by Billing & Sons, Worcester

Contents

Foreword

When issues are clearly and logically explored, we may be forgiven for thinking that they are simple and straightforward. This book can be seen as making complex situations more understandable by adopting different moral views during analysis. It sets out to provide an explanation of these views and shows how they lead to certain conclusions.

Not only is it fascinating to follow the logical argument used to discuss various dilemmas but also it is rather good fun. Using an interactive approach, Richard Rowson has seduced his readers into taking up the challenge not only to investigate their own views but also to apply other conventional moral standpoints.

Teamwork requires mutual respect and understanding. As staff become more aware of their differing priorities and opinions, they require the skills to analyse and explore problems and solutions. This book is a great contribution and should help nurses to enjoy the study of ethics and gain confidence in this important aspect of their work.

Jenifer Wilson-Barnett
Professor of Nursing Studies
King's College, London

Acknowledgements

I would like to thank the many people who encouraged and helped me in the writing of this book, most especially: Mary Armstrong, Kenneth Boyd, Paul Caine and students of Bulmershe College, Bridgit Dimond, Len Doyall, Ursula Gallagher, Evelyne Hide, Maureen Macmillan, Julian Mitchell, Rosemary Morris, Anthony O'Hear, Edward Shotter, Carolyne Sledmere, John Webb, Harvey White and Jenifer Wilson-Barnett.

RR

To my mother, Rita Anne Rowson, a student nurse at The London Hospital in the 1920s

Part 1

1 | Introduction

An Introduction to Ethics for Nurses is for everyone in nursing who wants to clarify their thinking about morality. 'Ethics', as used here, means 'thinking and reasoning about morality', and this book gives a concise explanation of the reasoning that lies behind the various moral attitudes we come across today.

Part 1 begins by sorting out some confusions you are likely to make when you first study morality. The various moral views that provide the basic elements of moral reasoning are then identified. They are explained with the aid of exercises, which require you to adopt the views and apply them to situations in nursing. In this way you can assess the merits of the various views and consider the part they play in your own moral thinking and in the thinking of your colleagues. There is then a brief consideration of the relationship between moral reasoning and personal feelings.

Part 2 begins by applying the moral views already examined to a difficult decision on the management of a patient. The case involves members of several health-care professions and shows how their different responsibilities can shape the way they see the moral issues. There are then further cases for you to consider, followed by a checklist of questions. This is to help you to identify all the moral issues you may need to think about in a difficult case. Finally, the professional Codes of Conduct are given so that you can consider them in the light of all the views you have looked at.

In writing this book I assume that all nurses wish to contribute fully to case conferences and interprofessional discussions, so are concerned to formulate their own views clearly and have an informed understanding of views that are different from their own.

I have tried to make the book as brief and straightforward as possible, since many nurses interested in thinking about morality do not want to study abstract theoretical matters or the history of moral thought. So, although the book deals with central issues of moral theory, it does so without discussing their theoretical context and without referring to key figures in their historical development. Readers who wish to delve more deeply are recommended to the books listed under 'Further reading'.

TIPS TO FOLLOW IN YOUR READING

Particularly important points are introduced by a bullet (●) and are set in **bold** type. Make sure you understand them. Here is one:

● **Understand a view before judging it.**

When some people start reading the sorts of idea discussed here, they try to do too much at once. *First* make sure you understand a view, *then* think about whether or not you agree with it. If you think about too much at once you will get confused.

You may want to read some sections slowly – or twice. If you are not used to thinking about moral issues, don't expect to read all of this book at the speed of a novel. New ideas take time to absorb.

Doing the exercises: The exercises are there to encourage you to think through the points in the text and sort out your own views. You will find it more interesting, and easier to remember what you think, if you jot down your responses to the exercises. You can then look back at them. You may find you are changing your mind! Writing thoughts down, if only for yourself, gives good practice at explaining your ideas.

Breaking up your reading: Reading books like this one tends to be more productive, and completed in less time, if you read when your concentration is fresh, so it is a good idea to take a break at suitable places: these are pointed out in the text.

WAYS IN WHICH WORDS ARE USED IN THIS BOOK

To avoid misunderstanding, here are some points about the way in which words are used in this book.

For simplicity, and to avoid constantly using the clumsy formula 'he or she' or the ugly and unpronounceable 's/he', nurses are generally referred to as 'she' and doctors and patients as 'he'. This is not an attempt to 'gender stereotype' roles in health care!

In ordinary conversation, 'moral' may be used in two ways:

1. to mean 'relevant to morality', as in:
   'How she treats her patients is a moral issue, but what colour she dyes her hair is not.'
2. to mean 'good', as in:
   'She's a very moral person and wouldn't shirk her responsibilities.'

It is very easy to confuse these two uses, but:

● **Whenever the word 'moral' is used in this book it is in the first sense – i.e. 'relevant to morality'.**

If 'good' or 'morally acceptable' is meant, these words are used.

● **'Ethics', as already pointed out, is used to mean 'thinking and reasoning about morality'.**

'Professional code' or 'professional etiquette' is used to mean 'the conventions of acceptable behaviour in the professions', such as the convention that only surgeons are addressed as 'Mr'.

2 | Judging from many standpoints

Every day we make judgments about what is 'right' or 'wrong', or what we 'ought' or 'ought not' to do. But not all of these judgments are made from a *moral* standpoint, as we can see from the following situations.

A nurse who is late going on duty knows it is *legally wrong* to exceed the speed limit. On the other hand, having delayed leaving home to help a neighbour who has had an accident, she thinks it is *morally right* to drive fast where it is safe to do so, as the ward she is working on is so short-staffed.

A Roman Catholic may believe that the use of condoms is wrong from a *religious* perspective, although he sees that, *practically*, they are good at reducing transmission of disease.

Although a nurse thinks it *looks wrong* to decorate a room in a jumble of designs, she thinks it is *morally right* if it cheers up the patients in a children's ward.

In these examples people make judgments about what is right and wrong from the standpoints of law, morality, visual taste and what is, in practical terms, effective. In fact, whatever our cultural and ethnic background, most of us from time to time judge behaviour from the standpoints of:

1. law;
2. social etiquette;
3. professional codes or professional etiquette;
4. religious beliefs;
5. our visual and 'aesthetic' sense;
6. what is most practical;
7. morality.

Briefly, we can say that:

1. The *legal* standpoint is about what is required and forbidden by the law of the country in which we live.

   e.g.: In the UK there is a legal obligation to report the fact that a patient's condition is the result of a terrorist incident. It is legally *wrong* not to do so.

2. *Social etiquette* applies accepted conventions to what some people regard as trivial aspects of behaviour.

   e.g.: In conventional British society it is *right* for a man to stand when a woman enters the room. In traditional Hindu society it is *right* for a woman to keep her head covered.

3. *Professional codes* and *professional etiquette* are concerned with governing conduct within a profession or between professions.

   e.g.: According to the UKCC Code of Professional Conduct, a nurse *ought* to refuse 'to accept delegated functions without first having received instruction in regard to those functions and having been assessed as competent'.

4. A *religious* standpoint sees humans as part of an overall divine scheme and judges behaviour on how it fits into that scheme.

   e.g.: For some Catholics it is *wrong* to use a condom for contraception because it interferes with what they see as the God-given purpose of sexuality.

5. *Visual* and *aesthetic* standpoints assess behaviour on whether or not it produces an effect that 'looks beautiful' or satisfies 'artistic sensitivity'.

   e.g.: Some people think it *wrong* aesthetically to decorate a room in a jumble of different designs and colours.

6. The *practical* standpoint considers whether actions are the most effective way of achieving whatever aim is in mind.

   e.g.: Practically, it is *wrong* to put an IV infusion in the right hand of a right-handed patient, if the patient is to be as independent as possible.

7. We shall look at what people think is the *moral* standpoint in the next section, where we shall find that there are very different views.

Not everyone agrees that there *is* a clear distinction between a moral standpoint and some of the other standpoints. For example, some people think that the morally right action in a situation is whatever action is the most effective practically, and some religious believers see no difference between their moral and their religious obligations, since they think that their moral obligation is to do whatever is God's will. Other religious believers, however, think that there is a difference between the two sorts of obligation. They would think, for example, that they have a religious, but not a moral, obligation to pray, and a moral, but not a religious, obligation to pay their train fare.

As you read on, you will have the opportunity to work out your views on these matters.

But let us note what we have seen so far:

● **We judge behaviour from several standpoints.**

● **We sometimes judge one action from several standpoints.**

● **We may judge an action right from one standpoint and wrong from another**.

Exercise 1

Bearing in mind the points just made, look at the actions below, then answer the questions.

1. A nurse calls a new patient, who is elderly, 'Sunny Jim' every time she talks to him.
2. A sister does not consult nurses before working out the holiday rota and sending it to the administrative department.
3. A Jehovah's witness refuses to let her daughter have a blood transfusion even though it is thought to be the only way to save her life.
4. An elderly lady is mentally sound but unable to look after herself. She does not want to leave her own home, but her daughter cannot look after her and cope with a young family. The daughter, doctor and district nurse pretend that she is being taken to hospital for two days for treatment, when in fact she is going to a home for the elderly, where they hope she will stay. They think that their action of pretending to her will cause her less distress than would telling her what is really going on.
5. The staff supervising mentally handicapped people in long-stay community care accommodation allow physical relationships to develop between residents of different sexes but try to prevent them between residents of the same sex.

continued next page

— Continued ——————————————————————

Questions

1. From which standpoints can each action be judged?
2. Do you think the actions are 'right' or 'wrong' from these standpoints?
3. What are your reasons for thinking that they are right or wrong?

You may find it quickest to jot down your answers under headings like this:

Action	Standpoint	Right/wrong, reasons
1. Calling the patient 'Sunny Jim'	Professional etiquette	Right/wrong because . . .
	Moral	Right/wrong because . . .

Do the exercise before reading on.

POINTS BROUGHT OUT BY DOING THE EXERCISE

Before considering possible responses to the exercise, let us look at some points that might have affected the way you responded.

You might have found that your personal beliefs affect the importance you give to some standpoints. For example, if you do not have any religious beliefs, you obviously could not judge *any* of the actions from this standpoint. On the other hand, if you have very strong beliefs from one standpoint, you might not have wanted to judge an action from any other. If, for example, you are a Jehovah's witness, you might see the mother's refusal of a blood transfusion only from the religious standpoint and regard all other standpoints as unimportant. So we see that:

● **Personal beliefs can affect the value you give to standpoints. They can, for example, prevent you judging actions from some standpoints, or can make you judge an action from only one standpoint**.

Before you could answer the questions in the exercise, you might have wanted more information about each situation. Without it, you may have had to guess what was 'really' going on.

Take the situation of the sister not consulting the nurses about the holiday rota. If you thought the sister was probably run off her feet just before the deadline to submit the rota, so that she had no opportunity to consult her colleagues, you might not have blamed her from a *moral* standpoint, although you might have thought she was *professionally* at fault. On the other hand, if you thought she had deliberately failed to speak to the nurses, then you might have thought she was *morally* wrong. This shows that:

● **Which standpoint you think is relevant to an action can depend on your interpretation of a situation.**

In the situation of the nurse calling the patient 'Sunny Jim', you might have wanted to know more about her intention or *motive*. Is she trying to raise his spirits or to assert her authority by making him feel childlike and subservient? So we see that:

● **Before you can decide whether an action is morally right or wrong, you may want to know about the motive behind it.**

You might also have wanted to know about the *effect* of an action. If the patient feels humiliated by being called 'Sunny Jim', does that make it wrong? If he feels more cheerful, does that make it right? So:

● **Before you can judge whether an action is morally right or wrong you may want to assess its likely effects.**

If you felt you needed more information about the motives or consequences of the actions before you could make your moral judgments, motives or consequences are obviously aspects of actions that are morally important for you.

● **For some people, morality is concerned with motives and/or consequences of actions.**

But are motives and consequences the only aspects of actions that may be important in morality? In the following responses to Exercise 1, other aspects of actions are also seen as morally important.

RESPONSES TO EXERCISE 1

These responses are not put forward as a 'correct' way of judging the actions. They are simply a set of possible responses. You may have thought of many others.

Action	Standpoint	Right/wrong, reason
1. Calling the patient 'Sunny Jim'	Social etiquette	*Wrong* – too informal
	Professional etiquette	*Wrong* – at least with new patients, according to the nursing process
	Moral	*Wrong* – if the motive is to humiliate the patient
		Right – if the motive is to make the patient feel at home
		Wrong – if the action is likely to humiliate the patient
		Right – if the patient is likely to feel more cheerful
		Wrong – if it shows no respect for patient.
2. Not consulting nurses	Professional etiquette	*Wrong* – nurses should be consulted over holidays
	Practical	*Wrong* – it will take more time and effort to sort out in the long run
	Moral	*Wrong* – inconsiderate of nurses' needs
3. Refusing blood	Religious belief	*Right* – from the mother's viewpoint of what is God's will
		Wrong – if we think it is God's will to save life by blood transfusions
	Moral	*Right* – if we think it morally most important that someone avoid what he sees as wrong
		Wrong – if we think it morally most important to save life

continued next page

Continued

4. Pretending to old lady	Legal	*Wrong* – it could be illegal to take a sane person somewhere without her permission
	Moral	*Wrong* – the action is dishonest: it is lying
		Wrong – the action is unjust as it takes unfair advantage of the old lady's weakness
		Wrong – the daughter, doctor and district nurse have a duty to respect the old lady's wishes
		Right – if it is likely to have better results than telling her the truth
5. Preventing only homosexual relationships	Moral	*Wrong* – does not respect the patients' wishes
		Wrong – unfair to restrict the freedom of some patients because of their sexual orientation
		Right – sexual relations between people of the same sex are unnatural
		Right – allowing such relationships to form is likely to lead to greater unhappiness and more problems in the long run

---

Exercise 2

1. Can you pick out the aspects of the actions that in these responses are thought to be *morally* important?
2. Are there other aspects of the actions that you think are morally important?

After thinking about answers to these questions, you may like to take a break.

3 Elements of ethics

Which aspects of actions people think are morally important shows the type of moral view that they hold. The list below gives the aspects picked out in the responses to Exercise 1 and the moral views that go with them. It is these views that are the basic elements in moral thinking or 'ethics'.

● **Morally important aspects of actions are:**

1. **when actions express attitudes to people.**
   Moral view:
   - Actions showing 'respect' and 'consideration' for people are morally right.
   - Actions showing 'disrespect' or 'lack of consideration' are morally wrong: e.g. in the examples above calling the patient 'Sunny Jim', and the sister failing to consult the nurses about the off–duty rota.

2. **when actions have certain qualities that make the actions right or wrong in themselves**.
   Moral view:
   - Qualities of honesty, justice or fairness make actions morally right.
   - Qualities of dishonesty, injustice or unfairness make actions morally wrong: e.g. in the examples above lying to the old lady, and treating patients differently because of their sexual orientation.

3. **when actions are likely to affect people in certain ways**.
   Moral view:
   - Actions likely to benefit people are morally right.
   - Actions likely to harm people are morally wrong: e.g. calling the patient 'Sunny Jim', and refusing the blood transfusion.

4. **when actions are done from certain motives**.
   Moral view:
   (a) – Concern to do or avoid certain types of action (e.g. dishonest or unfair actions) is the morally right motive.
   – Having no concern for doing or avoiding certain types of actions is morally wrong: e.g. lying to the old lady.

   or

   (b) – Concern to bring as much benefit as possible and as little harm as possible is the morally right motive.
   – Having no concern as to how actions affect people is morally wrong: e.g. sister not consulting the nurses.
5. **when actions are natural or unnatural.**
   Moral view:
   – Actions that are natural are morally right.
   – Actions that are unnatural are morally wrong: e.g. homosexual relationships.
6. **when actions agree with God's will or go against it**.
   Moral view:
   – Actions that are in agreement with God's will are morally right.
   – Actions that go against God's will are morally wrong: e.g. refusing or allowing the blood transfusion.

● **These views are the basic elements of moral thinking and they are held by people in various forms and combinations.**

Some people hold only one of the views and think that all moral decisions can be made on the basis of that view alone. Others think that more than one view must be adopted if all the morally important aspects of many situations are to be considered properly.

We shall consider each of these views in turn and, in the case study in the second part of this book, see how they can be applied to a particular situation.

As you look at each of the views you will be able to consider whether or not it is an element in your idea of morality. You will also be able to consider whether morality, as you see it, contains one, or several, of these elements.

RESPECTING PERSONS

We begin with the first view on page 13 that:

● **Actions showing respect for people are morally right and actions that 'use' people are morally wrong.**

What is it that makes having no respect for people, and 'using' people, so wrong? It may seem obvious to you that it *is* wrong, but can you explain why? Why is it acceptable to 'use' an object – say, a knife – but not a person – for example a nurse?

Exercise 3

Jot down what you think is a brief answer to the last question before reading on.

'Persons' have minds of their own. A nurse, for example, has knowledge of her surroundings and is aware of herself as a being with a future existence in which she has some choice as to what to do. Based on her understanding of her situation a person can:

1. think about what to do;
2. weigh up the pros and cons;
3. reach conclusions as to what she thinks is worthwhile;
4. form intentions and purposes;
5. make decisions;
6. carry out her decisions;
7. pursue objectives.

Knives, however, cannot do any of these things, and what is wrong about 'using' a person is that it treats her as though she cannot do any of them either. 'Respecting a person', on the other hand, gives her the opportunity to do all the things listed above: what is respected is her *right of self-determination* or *autonomy*, i.e. her capacity to 'rule' herself. ('Autonomy' is from the Greek *auto* = self and *nomos* = rule.)

Many people see respecting a mature person in this way as an essential part of morality, because only if a person is free to make up her own mind and act on her own decisions can she have moral responsibility for what she does. Someone who is not allowed this freedom is like a cog in a machine, which turns in a certain way because it is forced to do so by the other cogs. In this situation a person cannot be any more morally responsible than a cog.

In line with this view, to be fully morally responsible a mature person must not just carry out what she has been *told* are the right actions, without ever wondering whether or not she thinks they are right. This would make her no more morally responsible than a robot that has been programmed to operate in a certain way. To have moral goodness a mature person must decide for herself what to do and then act rightly of her own free will. If she does this, she has the human dignity of being an independent judge of what is right, and has the moral goodness of acting rightly voluntarily. But, obviously, none of this is possible if her autonomy is not respected. So we see that:

● **In this view, if you do not respect someone's personal autonomy (or right of self-determination), you do not allow them the freedom they need to be morally responsible for their actions.**

The right of self-determination is usually seen to include the right to act freely in several ways – such as to have freedom of speech, the freedom to mix with other people and the freedom to move unhindered about your own country.

Many people think that basic physical needs, and capacities for emotional and social relationships, are also essential parts of being a person, so we only 'respect the whole person' when we accept that someone has a right to satisfy these needs and capacities. In this view people have basic rights to warmth, food, shelter, and sexual, emotional and social life, and we should uphold these rights as part of our general moral obligation to respect persons.

The International Council of Nurses *Code for Nurses* (page 75) says that it is important for nurses to respect 'the rights of man'. This and the UKCC *Code of Professional Conduct* (page 65) talk of the need to respect the beliefs, values and customs of the individual.

Limits to 'respecting persons'

Someone who considers that respecting personal autonomy is essential to morality will still think that there are times when a person is entitled to tell others what to do and to make decisions on behalf of others.

There are many activities in health care – such as dealing with a cardiac arrest – that would be impossible to manage unless someone had the responsibility of organising others, and someone else carried out his orders. The leader of a cardiac arrest team is not seen as failing to respect the autonomy of other staff, and the staff are not seen as being 'used' by him. It is assumed that they have *chosen* to enter a career in which such situations occur, so have voluntarily given up their autonomy in such situations. But it does not, of course, follow from this that nurses are thought to have given up their autonomy in *all* professional situations.

As far as respecting the autonomy of the patient is concerned, it is normally thought morally right that a patient should give his informed consent to any treatment. This means that a patient's carers have a moral obligation to inform him as far as possible of the nature of his condition, of the alternative ways of treating him and of their likely side-effects and success rates. Only then can he give his 'informed' consent to any treatment. The Royal College of Nursing *Code of Professional Conduct Discussion Document* (page 68) says that 'the autonomy of the patient should be maintained throughout treatment, restrictions being imposed only when these are demonstrably necessary for [the patient's] own good'.

When patients are unable to understand their situation or express their thoughts as a result of accident, illness or disability, we obviously cannot respect their wishes. We must then stick to the guidelines of good practice. However, in cases such as dementia, where patients sometimes express their wishes, doctors, nurses, social workers and psychologists sometimes disagree as to how much the patient has 'a mind of his own'. How much should we respect the wishes of such a patient? In this type of case it may be useful to distinguish two meanings of 'having a mind of his own':

1. 'Knowing his *immediate desires*'.
2. 'Being able to *think out* his own decisions'.

A patient may have the former but not the latter. He may know, for instance, that he wants an apple and not an orange, but may not be able to think about the advantages and disadvantages of different forms of treatment. In such a case it may be morally right to respect his *immediate* desires as far as possible, while making decisions about his *long-term* treatment on his behalf.

DOING RIGHT ACTIONS AND AVOIDING WRONG ONES

(The 'dutiful' view)

We now turn to the second view on page 13 that:

● **Certain actions are right or wrong 'in themselves'. Morality is a matter of doing those actions that are right in themselves and avoiding those that are wrong in themselves.**

Actions may be seen as wrong in themselves because:

1. *they are actions that have certain qualities:*
   - qualities of honesty, truthfulness, fairness and justice make actions right in themselves;
   - deceit, unfairness or injustice make actions wrong in themselves;
2. *they are actions of a certain sort:*
   - e.g.: deliberately taking life, deliberate and unnecessary cruelty.

This is sometimes known as the *deontological* view (Greek, *deontos* = duty). We shall call it the *dutiful* view, because it considers that certain types of actions are our duties. Actions such as 'keeping promises', 'telling the truth', and 'being honest' are right in themselves and are *positive* duties. Actions such as 'not telling lies', 'not deceiving people', 'not being deliberately and unnecessarily cruel' and 'not deliberately taking life' are seen as *negative* duties. They ensure that we avoid actions that are wrong in themselves.

'Honesty' and 'truthfulness' basically mean 'not deceiving people'. 'Justice' and 'fairness' can mean one or all of the following:

1. *Regarding all people as equally valuable regardless of their age, sex, race, colour, sexual orientation, nationality and religious or political views.*

   It is 'fair' and 'just' to consider the well-being of each person as equally important, so treat everyone alike, unless there is some *relevant* difference between them that justifies treating them differently. For example, the different political views of people are not usually seen as relevant to the medical treatment they receive, but their different disabilities and medical needs are. This is why most people think it fair and just to ensure that people of all political parties have equal access to health-care facilities, but, of course, think that their different medical needs and disabilities justify giving them different treatment.

2. *Treating people impartially by applying rules or principles that are known and respected.*

It may, for example, seem 'unjust' or 'unfair' if a particular student is not reprimanded for an offence against hospital rules for which other students have been reprimanded. It may seem equally 'unjust' or 'unfair' if a student is reprimanded for doing something which none of the students knew to be against the rules.

3. *Treating people in a way they deserve, by giving them their 'just deserts', or by rewarding them 'according to their merit'.*

We may, for example, think it 'unfair' or 'unjust' if a nurse who is quite lazy is put forward for promotion before another who is very conscientious.

The foundation of morality?

Some people think that either 'respect for persons' or the 'dutiful view' is the foundation of all moral thinking.

Those who see the dutiful view as the foundation of morality consider that their convictions that certain actions are right or wrong in themselves are the most basic moral convictions they have. They think that all their other ideas about morality are built on these 'gut' convictions. So, for them it is impossible to explain *why* certain actions are right or wrong, because they have no convictions that are *more* fundamental which could support or justify them.

Those who see 'respect for persons' as the foundation on which all their ideas about morality are built claim that they *can* explain why certain acts are regarded as right or wrong in themselves. They think that acts of honesty, fairness and justice are right *because* they show respect for people, and acts of dishonesty, unfairness and injustice, deliberate killing and cruelty are wrong *because* they do not value or respect people. In their view, if someone lies to you, he is reducing your capacity to understand your surroundings; and since this capacity is a valuable part of you as a person, he is thus failing to respect you as a person and is manipulating or 'using' your intelligence for his own purposes.

Exercise 4

1. Do you have basic convictions that are the foundation on which all your other moral ideas are built?
   If so, jot down what they are.
2. Do you think that any of the following is the foundation of morality?:
   – respect for personal autonomy;
   – the moral duty to do actions that are right 'in themselves'; and avoid those that are wrong 'in themselves';
   – a combination of these factors;
   – some other factor not yet discussed?

This is a good place to take a break.

SEEKING THE BEST CONSEQUENCES

(The 'utilitarian' view)

This is the third view on page 13. It is the view that:

● **Morally right actions are those which are the most useful in producing the best consequences for everyone.**

Since this view considers that actions only have moral value if they are *useful*, it is known as the *utilitarian* view (utility = usefulness).

Utilitarians think that it is our moral obligation to try to produce the best consequences we can. They have put forward various ideas as to what they mean by 'the best consequences', for example:

1. the greatest amount of *pleasure* and the smallest amount of pain or *suffering* possible;
2. the greatest amount of *happiness* and the least amount of *unhappiness* possible;
3. the greatest amount of human and animal *well-being* possible.

These are attempts to describe the ideal that they think we should aim for if we want to act morally well. Utilitarians admit that we cannot ever know whether the actions we carry out have actually achieved the best consequences possible, since we cannot be certain what would have happened if we had acted differently. But they think that it is valuable to have a 'picture' of an ideal, which it is our moral obligation to strive after when we are deciding how to behave. (Ideal 'pictures' play a similar role in other views. In Christianity, for example, Christ's life can be seen as providing an ideal to strive after, rather than as something that can actually be achieved.)

For utilitarians, when a person has a chance to choose what to do, his moral obligation is to look at all the possible courses of action open to him and assess the likely benefit and harm of each course of action on everyone affected.

When doing this he should regard greater benefits as more valuable than smaller ones, and should regard everyone as *equally* important. So, if a benefit on someone unconnected to him is greater than the benefit on someone close to him, he should consider the effect on the remote person as more valuable. In this way the utilitarian approach to making moral decisions rules out selfishness or concern only for one's own family or community. Utilitarians also think that a morally responsible person should be concerned with *all* the likely effects of his actions, so should think about long-term as well as immediate consequences.

When someone has assessed, as sincerely and thoroughly as he can, all the likely effects of all the actions open to him, he should try to act in the way he thinks will produce the best consequences. Only when he has carried out this process to the best of his ability has he fulfilled his moral obligation. So, when a doctor is deciding how to manage a patient he should assess the immediate and long-term benefits and harms of all the alternative treatments on the patient, his family, his friends and the nurses involved in the patient's care.

Many utilitarians claim that although we cannot always go through this process every time we try to act morally well, we should try to carry it out whenever we can, as it is morally the ideal way to make a decision.

Exercise 5

Do you think this process *is* the morally ideal way to make decisions, when there is time to do so?

As we do not have time to go through the ideal process every time we have to make a decision, many utilitarians think we need rules of thumb about how to behave, which we can refer to when in a hurry. These rules are decided upon by working out which types of action would in *most* circumstances be likely to bring greatest benefit to everyone in the long run.

Some people think that, in fact, many of our traditional principles and ideas about morality – e.g. principles of fairness and axioms like 'keep your promises' and 'don't tell lies' – are really utilitarian guidelines. They think that they are conclusions that people have reached over the centuries as to how it is best to behave in most circumstances in order to benefit society in the long run. They see these rules as guidelines, which should be followed when we are in a hurry, but which we do not have to stick to when we have time to do a careful assessment of our particular circumstances. So, if we sincerely think on a particular occasion that we are likely to bring about better consequences by breaking a rule, then it is our moral obligation to break it, and do whatever we honestly think is likely to cause the greatest amount of benefit over harm in the circumstances. Holders of such views see no moral value in rules or in any particular type of action. For them rules such as 'keep promises', or actions like telling the truth, have moral value only when they are likely to produce more benefit than would other actions. Only in such circumstances are we morally obliged to perform them.

The following situation illustrates this view and also brings out the contrast between the utilitarian and 'dutiful' views of morality.

A nurse, John, takes a utilitarian approach to morality. He thinks, for example, that it normally brings greatest benefit to everyone if people keep their promises.

One day, Anne, a close colleague is very depressed and tells him that her husband told her the previous evening that he wants to end their marriage. She is unable to concentrate on her work or take any interest in the patients. She doesn't want the other staff to know about her problems and John promises to keep it to himself.

The next day Anne makes a mistake in the medication of a patient and the sister is furious with her. The sister has high professional standards but she tends to be resentful of the younger female nurses like Anne. She will bear a grudge about her mistake and complain about it for a long time.

John thinks it will be very damaging to Anne if she is the victim of the sister's continuing resentment. It will only make Anne more tense and likely to make more mistakes. He thinks that if the sister knew the truth she would drop the matter. He honestly thinks that greatest benefit will be brought to all concerned if he breaks his promise and tells the sister in confidence what has happened. So he sees it as his *moral obligation* to tell the sister about Anne's marital problems. He does not think it is at all wrong to break his promise, since promise-keeping has no value in itself for him.

However, if John held the dutiful view of morality he would consider that breaking a promise is an action that is *wrong* in itself. He would see it as his moral duty to keep his promise and not let his concern for Anne stop him from doing his duty.

HAVING THE RIGHT MOTIVE

Let us now turn to the fourth view on page 14, which is the idea that morality is concerned with the motives behind actions. There are two views about moral motivation and they are really part of the dutiful and utilitarian views.

1. ● **Moral motivation is concern to do the right actions and avoid the wrong ones**.

This is the view that we are only motivated by morality when we are concerned to do actions that are right in themselves and avoid those that are wrong in themselves, so is part of the dutiful view.

● **The dutiful view claims that**:
   – morality is a matter of carrying out our **duty** to perform or avoid actions that are right or wrong in themselves;
   – the motivation to act morally is the concern to do actions because they are right, and not for any other reason. This is sometimes summed up as **'duty for duty's sake'**;
   – morality is its **own reward**.

According to this view, if we are motivated by morality, we will want to be honest, for example, because honesty is morally right in itself and so is our duty, and *not* because honesty may lead to something else we value – such as the admiration of our friends. For if we were to act honestly in order to be admired we would not be motivated by morality at all, but by expediency, as we would really be concerned to bring about the consequences we wanted, and not with our moral *duty*. We would only value honesty because it happened to be useful, and not because of the value that honest actions have in themselves. So we would be ignoring their true moral value.

In this way the dutiful view sees concern to do or avoid actions that are right or wrong in themselves as the only *truly moral* motivation. Any other motivation has no moral value.

2. ● **Moral motivation is concern to bring about the best consequences**.

The utilitarian view of moral motivation is in sharp contrast to the dutiful view. According to the utilitarian view, we are only *morally* motivated when we are concerned to make our actions as useful as possible by bringing about the best consequences we can. In this view, no other motivation has moral value.

● **The utilitarian view claims that**:
   – moral motivation is concern to bring about the best **consequences**;
   – morality is not its 'own reward': the value of morality is the **benefits** that it may produce.

You can often see the difference between the dutiful and utilitarian views of moral motivation when people discuss euthanasia. People who have a dutiful view of moral motivation think that we should avoid doing any action that is wrong in itself. So, in discussion they will be mainly concerned with whether or not euthanasia is an act of deliberate killing, which they see as wrong 'in itself'. If they decide it is such an act, they will regard euthanasia as morally wrong.

On the other hand, those who have a utilitarian view of moral motivation think that we should be concerned to act in whatever way is likely to lead to the least pain and suffering, so they may look more favourably on euthanasia and see it as morally right in certain circumstances.

Exercise 6

Consider your view of moral motivation. When you make a decision, do you think you should be concerned with:
1. which actions are right or wrong in themselves;
2. which actions are likely to lead to the best consequences;
3. both the above factors;
4. some other concern not yet discussed?

Many people think that moral motivation involves both (1) and (2) above. They think it would be irresponsible to be concerned only with the rightness and wrongness of the actions themselves and to ignore their likely consequences. They also think it would be wrong to concentrate only on the consequences and not be concerned about the types of action needed to achieve them, for, if you are not concerned with the types of action you carry out, you might honestly think on rare occasions that, if some horrific act is the only way to bring about a very valuable consequence, you ought to carry it out. In an extreme situation you might decide, for example, that you ought to kill a healthy older person because transplanting his organs is the only way to save the lives of several younger people.

Considerations such as these have led some people to think that neither the dutiful view nor the utilitarian view alone gives an adequate description of moral motivation. They have concluded that what is needed is a combination of these views.

A combined view

When reading about the dutiful and utilitarian views you too may have wondered whether there is any way of reconciling them, since you may feel they both have a part to play in morality. Let us look at this possibility.

● **One 'combined' view is that, although certain actions are right or wrong in themselves, their rightness and wrongness has to be weighed against their consequences.**

In this view the rightness or wrongness of the actions will sometimes outweigh the value of their likely consequences. At other times the value of the consequences will outweigh the rightness or wrongness of the actions. A person's moral obligation is to consider the value of both actions and consequences, and go for the greater value.

Let us look again at John's situation on page 22.

If John had held this combined view, he would be faced with a moral dilemma, for he would think both that it is wrong to break a promise and that he ought to benefit everyone as much as possible. He would then have to use his knowledge of the situation to weigh the wrongness of breaking his promise against the likely benefit and harm of doing so.

From his knowledge of the sister he might think, for example, that she would keep the information confidential and handle the situation tactfully, so the benefit of breaking the promise would outweigh the wrongness of it. On this basis he would decide that *in these circumstances* it is morally right to break the promise, although he regrets having to do it as he still thinks breaking promises is wrong.

We now see how the combined view differs from the utilitarian one. As a utilitarian, John had no regrets about breaking a promise, because he did not see anything wrong in promise-breaking as an act itself.

What if John held the 'combined' view, but his knowledge of the situation was different and he thought that Anne would realise from the sister's behaviour that he had broken his promise? This would make Anne even more depressed because she would feel betrayed. In these circumstances he would think the consequences would certainly *not* outweigh the wrongness of breaking his promise, so he ought to keep it.

From this example we see that the combined view involves more complex considerations than either the dutiful or utilitarian view alone. Some people see this as a disadvantage of the combined view. Others, however, think that the combined view includes elements from both views that are essential for making moral decisions that take into account the complexity of many 'real life' situations.

Exercise 7

Consider the following situations:

1. You are a psychiatric nurse who for several weeks has given support to a depressed client, Jane. She is gradually regaining her self-esteem and, as the one thing she thinks she can do is cook rather well, she has the idea of giving you a treat by cooking you a meal. You realise that it is important for her to feel she can do something for you. Unfortunately, you don't enjoy the meal – far too much black pepper in the main course, the pudding not sweet enough and the wine too acidic. She asks you whether you have enjoyed the meal.

2. As part of her recovery Jane goes out alone to buy a new outfit and returns, very pleased with herself, to show it to you. You think the colours she has chosen make her look ill, and the fit doesn't flatter her figure. She asks you whether you like it.

Briefly outline how you would think about these situations if you adopted:

– the combined view;
– the dutiful view;
– the utilitarian view.

RESPONSES TO EXERCISE 7

If you adopt the *combined* view, these situations give you a moral dilemma because you think both that it is wrong to tell lies and that you have a moral obligation to benefit Jane as much as possible. As you cannot satisfy both moral demands, you have to weigh one against the other.

In (1) you may decide that the wrongness of telling a lie is much less important than the harm it will do Jane if you tell her the truth, since this would make her think that her first attempt to do something constructive is a failure. You may think that she is unlikely to find out later that you were lying, since you can easily keep up the pretence. So you decide it is morally right to tell a lie. You *regret* having to do it, as you think it is wrong to tell lies, but you are certain you are morally *justified* in doing so *in these circumstances*.

In (2), however, you may think that, although lying to Jane will boost her confidence at that moment, she will later be likely to realise, or be told by others, that the clothes do not suit her, and this would be worse for her in the long run. Also, the situation is retrievable, since she can change the clothes – but in (1) you cannot eat another meal! So you decide that in circumstance (2) it is right to tell the truth. You *regret* causing Jane some unhappiness, but you think you are *justified* in doing so *in this particular situation*.

If you adopt the *dutiful* view you may think that, since lying is an action that is wrong in itself, you should tell the truth in both situations. Although you may feel unhappy about the misery Jane may experience, you do not think it is morally wrong to cause it.

In this view there is a difference between *feeling* happy or sad about what may happen as a result of your actions, and *judging* that your actions are right or wrong – and holders of the dutiful view think the two should not be confused. They see the first as an emotional response, which is irrelevant to morality.

We shall come back to this view in chapter 4, 'Morality and personal feelings', in which we shall look at various opinions on the relationship between emotions and moral judgments.

If you adopt the *utilitarian* view, you may think that in (1) you should tell a lie, since this would be likely to bring most benefit – but you would not feel any regret at all about having lied, because you see nothing wrong about lying in itself.

In (2) you may think you should tell the truth – not because there is anything right about truth-telling in itself, but because in these particular circumstances it is likely to bring about the best consequences.

Exercise 8

1. How much are you in agreement with responses of each of the three views?
2. Do people around you ever adopt lines of argument similar to any of the above when they are faced with moral decisions?

If you want a rest, this is a good place to take a break.

Let us now turn to the fifth view on page 14 – 'acting naturally' and 'doing God's will'.

ACTING IN ACCORD WITH NATURE

Many people who see some acts as 'natural' and others as 'unnatural' regard 'unnatural' acts as wrong.

● **Actions that are 'unnatural' are wrong.**

The connection between 'wrong' and 'unnatural' is so strong in some people's minds that to say that something is unnatural is often enough to condemn it. Someone who says, 'It's unnatural for a boy to play with dolls' implies that such behaviour is wrong.

The view that 'unnatural' acts are wrong obviously relies on being able to make a distinction between 'natural' and 'unnatural' acts. How this distinction is made depends on whether the term 'nature' is thought to mean:

1. 'nature as a whole' – the system of nature; or
2. 'human nature'.

If 'nature' is used to mean 'nature as a whole' or 'the system of nature' then:

'natural' = 'in accord with the system of nature'
'unnatural' = 'interferes with the system of nature; artificial'
e.g. 'Herbal remedies are the natural treatment.'
    'Spare part surgery is unnatural.'

When people use these words in this way their view seems to be that *any* interference with nature is wrong. But can that really be their view? We constantly interfere with nature whenever we use our intelligence to control or improve our natural environment – where we live, what we eat and how we deal with disease. If you look at the actions listed in Exercise 9 below, you will see that nearly all interfere with nature to a greater or lesser extent.

Indeed, since most of our everyday actions do interfere with nature, it is difficult to claim that *all* actions that do so are wrong. To make such a claim one would have to be prepared to say that humans should not use their intelligence to control nature at all – and no-one takes that line of argument.

As no-one regards *all* interference with nature as wrong, it cannot be the simple fact that nature is interfered with that makes an action 'unnatural' and wrong in this view. So what is it that makes some interferences 'unnatural' but not others? Is it 'natural' to interfere with nature up to a certain point but not beyond it? Exercise 9 will help you think about these questions.

Exercise 9

Where do you make the distinction between 'natural' and 'unnatural' actions in the following?:

1. Living in – a high rise, air–conditioned flat;
   – a centrally heated, double–glazed house;
   – a mud hut with thatched roof;
   – a cave.
2. Eating – food containing chemically produced preservatives and additives;
   – food containing refined sugar and flour;
   – food that has been cooked;
   – food that has been washed but not cooked;
   – food that has been picked but not washed.
3. Treating by – high-tech surgery;
   – cutting with a knife;
   – chemically produced medicines;
   – herbal medicines;
   – bathing in boiled water;
   – bathing in cold water.

This exercise shows how difficult it is to claim that interference with nature is 'natural' up to a certain level, but 'unnatural' beyond it. For at what point can we fix the level? Look at the following suggestions.

1. Sometimes people talk as though everything in nature has *one* particular purpose, and that an unacceptable level of interference has been reached when something is used for a purpose that is different from its particular one.

● **In this view it is 'natural' (so right) to use something for its particular purpose, but 'unnatural' (so wrong) to use it for any other.**

This view assumes that we can know what is *the* particular purpose of something. But can facts of nature alone make this clear to us? Or is what we regard as *the* purpose of something simply the purpose for which we traditionally use it?

Take salt and water, for instance. Can we really claim that what we know about salt shows that the purpose of it is, say, to enhance the flavour of food, and what we know about water tells us that the purpose of it is to quench thirst – so are we misusing salt and water when we use them for any other purpose, as in a saline drip? The more we have learned about salt and water, the more uses we have found for them, so it is impossible to identify, from the facts of nature alone, which is *the* purpose for them.

2. At other times people talk of things in nature having a *number* of proper purposes.

● **In this view it is right to use something for its 'proper purposes' and wrong to use it for any others.**

Again, it is difficult to find any factual basis in nature for this view: where to draw the line, for instance, between 'proper' and 'improper' uses of water. We cannot answer this question by looking at the facts of nature alone, for they indicate hundreds of uses for water.

Surely, the facts of nature simply show us that most natural things have many qualities and can be used in many different ways. Humans have always applied their intelligence to finding new facts about nature and have constantly discovered new ways of using nature. So it seems that what people think of as *the* purpose, or the 'proper' purpose, of something is simply the purpose for which that thing has *normally* been used in *their* experience.

3. There are also people who talk of nature as having intentions: 'Nature never intended . . . ' they say, or, 'If nature had intended . . . .':

    e.g. 'Nature never intended men to go to the moon.'

       'If nature had intended women to be cool, rational creatures, they would not have been made victims of the menstrual cycle.'

● **In this view it is right to use nature in accordance with 'nature's intentions', and wrong to go against these intentions.**

As with the two previous views, it is difficult to see how the facts of nature alone justify this view. Might it not be, for example, that nature intended humans to use their intelligence to work out how to get to the moon? What facts can we pick out that clearly show that nature did or did not intend this? And could we not pick out another set of facts that would indicate something different?

If the views of people who see nature as having intentions are explored further, it usually turns out that they do not actually rely on facts of nature alone to identify these intentions. They generally also hold religious or other theoretical beliefs, and it is these beliefs, and not just the facts of nature, that make them see nature as having certain intentions.

This is not really surprising, because we normally think of intentions as belonging to people and not to things; that is, we usually regard 'intentions' as being ideas in someone's *mind*. So, when people talk of nature having 'intentions', it is likely that they will see nature either as having a mind of its own or as having been designed by a mind – or a God – who *intends* nature to act in a certain way. Many Roman Catholics, for example, consider that human sexuality is a part of nature intended to be used within marriage for the production of children. For them, to use sex in other ways is to misuse it. Behind this view lies the idea that God has given us our sexuality, and it is His intention that we should use sex only in this way.

So, when people say 'Nature never intended us to use . . . in that way', this really amounts to saying 'According to my particular beliefs, we ought not to use nature in that way.'

We have seen, then, that people who say that certain actions are wrong because they interfere with the system of nature do not disapprove of all actions that interfere with nature, but only with those that do so in ways they do not like, or are not used to, or which do not fit in with their religious or theoretical standpoint. Their claim that certain acts are wrong because they are 'unnatural' is deceptive because it is not based on the facts of nature alone: they have other reasons for disapproving of the actions.

However if by 'nature' is meant 'human nature', then:

'natural' = 'in accordance with human nature'
'unnatural' = 'goes against human nature'
e.g. 'It's only natural for the old lady to want to stay in her own
home.'
'It's unnatural to bring children up in a kibbutz.'

● **In this view, what is in accord with human nature is right;
what goes against human nature is wrong.**

This can only be an effective guide to acting rightly if we can
identify human nature sufficiently precisely to say which actions are in
accordance with human nature and which are not.

But there are many different aspects to our nature: physical desires,
instincts, emotions, rationality and intellectual aspirations. They are
sometimes at war with each other, but as they are all parts of human
nature, how can we say that acting in accord with one of them is more
true to human nature than acting in accord with another?

People sometimes say that physical desires – for food and sex for
example – and emotions – such as love and hate – are more 'basic' and
fundamental parts of our nature than are our powers of reasoning, so
we should follow them. But other people think that higher level
reasoning is what distinguishes human from animal nature, so to be
true to human nature we should follow reasoning rather than desire.

Sometimes people say that the most 'natural' way to behave is to act
spontaneously, but the problem with that idea is that we often think
we have acted wrongly when we have acted spontaneously. 'If only I
had thought about it a bit more!' we say, showing that, far from
simply going along with our spontaneous reactions, we think we
should be wary of them. When we have time to stop and think our
considered moral judgments are often not the same as our immediate
reactions.

Moreover, if someone thinks that the guide to acting rightly is 'act
spontaneously', what guidance can he offer to someone who has no
spontaneous response to a situation? When a doctor or nurse is
agonising as to whether or not to give a very heavy dose of painkilling
drugs to a terminally ill patient, it is no help to suggest to them that
they 'act spontaneously'.

Other people claim that certain actions are 'unnatural' and wrong
on the grounds that, as the majority of people do not do them, they
must be against human nature. For example:

'It's unnatural for – a boy to play with dolls';
           – people of the same sex to make love';
           – first cousins to marry'.

However, people who think in this way do not label as 'unnatural' and wrong all activities that the majority do not do – such as writing symphonies, performing brain operations or being celibate. So, the mere fact that an action is performed by a minority does not seem to be their actual reason for regarding it as wrong, but a reason they use to give added support to a view that they already hold for other reasons.

In this section we have seen the difficulty of finding, in the facts of nature alone, any basis for labelling actions 'natural' or 'unnatural'. An appeal to what is, or is not, 'in accord with nature' (whether by 'nature' is meant 'nature as a whole' or 'human nature') does not by itself give a guide to acting rightly.

DOING GOD'S WILL

We now look at the final view identified on page 14. For many people:

● **Right actions are those which are in agreement with God's will and wrong actions are those which go against God's will.**

In this short book we cannot explore particular views of God's will, since it would involve going into too many details of religious traditions. All we can do is notice one or two points about the general view that morality is based on God's will, and about the relationship between religious and non-religious moral views.

God's will as to how humans should behave is believed to be revealed in several different ways.

One view is that God's will is expressed in a set of statements in a sacred book – such as the Ten Commandments in the Bible. In this view acting rightly is a matter of obediently following rules or of learning how to apply rules. However, there may be different opinions as to how such rules should be applied to particular circumstances, especially to the new situations that occur in health care.

Another view is that God's will is revealed in examples of ideal behaviour – such as the lives and actions of Christ and the Saints.

Morality involves interpreting how to apply these examples to the circumstances of individual lives. Again, there may be different views on how to interpret them.

A third view is that God's will is revealed directly to individuals through their personal relationship with God. Although there may sometimes be dispute as to how to understand direct revelations, many believers think that God makes very clear to them what they should do in particular situations, so for them there is no scope for disagreement or discussion.

Given that there are different ways in which God's will is believed to be revealed, it is not surprising that people from different religious traditions, and sometimes within the same tradition, disagree as to what exactly is God's will and how it should be applied in particular circumstances. So we find that, although most religions believe that to live according to God's will we should value life and not deliberately destroy it, there are different opinions as to whether or not there can ever be exceptions to these general principles – for example, whether life may be taken in a just or Holy war, or whether euthanasia is ever permissible. So we see that:

● **Agreement to act in accordance with God's will does not always produce agreement about what should be done in particular circumstances.**

Of course, disagreement does not only occur among people who base their morality on God's will. People who share the same non-religious moral view, such as utilitarians, often disagree as to how their principles should be applied to particular circumstances.

Let us now turn to the relationship between those moral views that are based on God's will and those that are not.

Sometimes people who have a God-based morality agree with non-religious people about what should be done in particular circumstances. For example, a Muslim and a utilitarian may agree that life-prolonging treatment should not be given to a terminally ill patient. But even though they agree on what ought to be done, they will have different reasons for reaching their conclusions. The Muslim may reach his conclusion mainly because he thinks that to attempt to delay imminent death is going against the will of God, whereas the utilitarian thinks that treatment should be withheld because it would increase the suffering of the patient. Moreover, if the utilitarian has no belief in God, he will not see the Muslim's reason as a good reason for withholding treatment, for a non-believer cannot see there is any moral obligation to conform to the wishes of a Being he thinks does not exist.

A similar situation may occur between people who hold two non-religious moral views. They, too, might agree about what ought to be done, but for different reasons. For example, someone with a dutiful view of morality might think a patient should be told the truth about his terminal condition because telling the truth is 'good in itself', whereas a utilitarian might think that the truth should be told because in this particular case more benefit would come from telling the truth than from telling a lie. Again, although they agree on what ought to be done, they would not accept each other's reason as a good reason for making the decision. The utilitarian could not accept that telling the truth was 'good in itself', for he sees something as good only if it brings benefits. Equally, the dutiful person could not accept that a particular action is good simply because it brings benefits.

These two examples show us that:

● **What is a good reason for doing something in one moral view may not be a good reason in another moral view.**

● **The fact that an action is believed to be in accordance with the will of God does not give a non-believer a moral obligation to carry it out.**

So, when a religious believer claims that something ought to be done because it is God's will, he should realise that this does not give a good reason for doing it to someone who genuinely does not believe in God. The non-believer, in turn, should also realise that, if believers see an action as being in accordance with God's will, this *does* give them a good reason to carry it out, and he should respect their point of view.

When thinking about the relationship between moral views that are based on God's will and those which are not, people often question whether non-believers can have as firm a foundation for their moral views as believers.

Some people consider that a person who has no belief in God cannot have any basis on which to make moral judgments, for they see belief in God as giving humans their sense of right and wrong, and as inspiring them to seek moral perfection.

Others consider that a non-believer *can* have moral principles and ideals that give him as firm a basis as a believer for his moral judgment. They would, for example, consider that a utilitarian who makes a careful assessment of the likely consequences of using contraceptive devices, and concludes that it is right to use them, can have just as well-considered a basis for his moral judgment, and be just as morally conscientious, as a Catholic who considers contraceptives are wrong because they make humans misuse sexuality.

Exercise 10

Do you think that non-believers can have as firm a foundation as believers for their moral views?

REVIEW

We have now looked at all the views identified on pages 13 and 14 as the basic elements in moral thinking. On page 14 I wrote:

> Some people hold only one of the views and think that all moral decisions can be made on the basis of that view alone. Others think that more than one view must be adopted if all the morally important aspects of many situations are to be considered properly.
>
> As you look at each of the views you will be able to consider whether or not it is an element in your idea of morality. You will also be able to consider whether morality, as you see it, contains one, or several, of these views.

Exercise 11

1. Think about your idea of morality.

Are any of the views we have looked at elements in your idea of what morality is? If so, which?

2. Think about the views of people you know and work with.

Can you pick out any of these views in the moral opinions they express? Do you know people who stick to only one of these moral views? Do you know people who combine more than one moral view?

4 Morality and personal feelings

So far we have not considered emotions and personal feelings in relation to morality.

Exercise 12

Imagine that you read about a terrorist attack on a hospital in a town you frequently visit, in which several patients are killed. Then imagine that you read about a similar attack on a hospital in which roughly the same number of patients die, but which takes place in a part of the world you know very little about and do not expect to visit.

Do you think there would be any difference in your *emotional* reactions to each situation? Do you think that one attack is *morally worse* than the other?

It is likely that your emotions would be more affected by the attack in the area you visit than the one in the part of the world you know little about. However, you might think that morally the attacks are equally wrong. Similarly, you might be much more upset if a member of your family suffered a great deal of pain through poor terminal care than if someone you do not know suffered the same amount of pain in a similar situation. But you might consider the two situations equally wrong morally.

Many people think that such examples show that personal feelings are quite different from moral judgments. They see personal feelings as urging us to act in a particular way because of our *individual reactions* to particular people or situations, whereas they see our moral judgments as the result of *impartial reasons*.

Such reasons may be, for example, the moral requirement that we respect the autonomy of others, or that we seek the best consequences.

People who consider we should respect autonomy think we should show this respect to everyone impartially and not just to those we happen to like. And people who believe that we should seek the best consequences think we should regard everyone's well-being as being of equal moral value, regardless of our personal feelings towards them as individuals. In the example of poor terminal care they would consider it just as important morally to try to obtain better terminal care for the people we do not know as for the people we do.

This view of morality as impartial is put forward in the RCN *Code of Professional Conduct discussion document,* which considers that nurses ought not to let their personal feelings towards patients influence the quality of care they give:

> 'At times nurses may have prejudices against patients or clients . . . But the adoption of a professional attitude requires that all those who require nursing care should receive it without discrimination.'

Many people who see moral reasons as different from personal feelings in this way still regard feelings as morally important: they think that when we decide how to act, we should always take into account our own and other people's feelings and the likely effects of our actions on these feelings.

Of course, not everyone agrees that moral judgments *are* different from personal feelings. Someone who thinks, for example, that we should be true to nature by acting spontaneously is likely to think that the different degrees of affection and aggression we feel for individuals should decide how we treat them. But while this view may be appealing at first sight, just think what might happen if the strong feelings for each other that we sometimes experience were allowed to go unchecked by any impartial considerations!

In most major religions there are varying views on the role that feelings should play. In Buddhism, Christianity, Hinduism, Islam and Judaism there are sects that induce strong feelings in their members. These emotions – such as devotion, humility, love, anger, courage and bravery – are seen as an acceptable spur to right behaviour. But in the same religious traditions there are also groups who think that it is valuable to control emotions through calm and deliberate exercise of the mind. Some use reasoning to work out principles and codes of conduct to live by, as they think it is better for them to live according to the conclusions of reasoning than follow the impulses of feelings. Others use meditation or similar techniques to free themselves from emotions and desires, because they think that these desires prevent them from developing the calm state of mind they need to perceive the right way to live.

Exercise 13

How much do your personal feelings and emotions influence you when you are deciding what you ought to do?

Do you think you ought to be influenced by your feelings and emotions more or less than you are?

To be morally aware of a situation do you think a person needs to think about:

1. the different moral views that people may have in the situation?
2. the different personal feelings and emotions that people may have?

Before going on to Part 2, you may want to take a break.

Part 2

5 A case study

In this case study we explore ways in which the moral views that we have looked at in Part 1 apply to a particular situation. The case is a fairly complex one and we shall look at the points of view of everyone involved in the situation – patient, family, relatives, nurses, doctors, resource managers and administrators. How much each should be taken into account is a matter for you to consider.

MRS GREEN

Mrs Green, aged 61, was brought into hospital with severe chest pains and breathing difficulties. She also found it hard to swallow. When she was given an endoscopy she stopped breathing and was resuscitated, but after that her breathing remained weak.

A week later her breathing became so inadequate that it was necessary to put her on a ventilator. At this stage there was no clear diagnosis.

Subsequent tests have shown she has motor neurone disease and that she is unlikely to breathe again on her own. She has lost her ability to swallow, is not able to speak and is in pain and constant discomfort. However, she remains fully alert and is thinking clearly. She writes sensible notes to the medical staff, her husband, family and friends who visit her regularly, and she seems to be coping fairly well with the level of pain.

Her prognosis is not good. She will be prone to chest infections, which will become fatal if not treated. Her faculties will deteriorate at an unpredictable rate and her condition will become increasingly painful.

There seem to be three choices for her management:

1. She is kept on the ventilator and given full life-prolonging treatment – all infections will be treated, etc. With this treatment she could live for another 18 months, with her faculties deteriorating. She would be subject to repeated infections, increasingly invasive treatment and increasing pain. This is seen as the option that will cause the greatest amount of suffering but also the greatest prolongation of Mrs Green's life.

2. She is kept on the ventilator but not given life-prolonging treatment. Should an infection arise she will not be given antibiotics but kept as comfortable as possible until she succumbs to the infection. This would be likely to happen in 3 to 4 months. She would be in increasing discomfort, gradually deteriorating. This form of management is likely to give her less suffering than the previous course of action, but also a shorter life.

3. She is given treatment to make her comfortable and taken from the ventilator to see if she can breathe without it. She might be able to do so, but it is unlikely that this would last more than a few hours. She would be kept continually comfortable until her breathing ceased. This is the form of management likely to give her the least suffering, but also the shortest life expectancy.

Exercise 14

Before reading on, jot down what, at this moment, you think ought to be done in this case. Try to explain the reasons for your decision. Later you can look back at your response and compare it with the other views we shall look at.

Let us first look at some of the personal feelings that may arise in the case.

PERSONAL FEELINGS

Whether or not Mrs Green is made aware of her prognosis, her feelings may vary enormously. At one extreme she may feel panic and fear at what she either knows or suspects may lie ahead. She may have no interest in continuing her life, want to escape the prospect of further pain and hope to be given an early and painless death. At the other extreme she may very much want to live as fully as she can for as long as she can.

The people who spend most of the time with Mrs Green are her husband, relatives, friends and the nursing staff. They may feel love or fondness for her, sadness at her disability and admiration at the way she has coped so far. They will also be affected by her feelings, insofar as they know them. If they think that she is fearful and hoping for a painless and early death, some may want her wishes to be met. If, on the other hand, they think she wants to live as fully as possible, they may hope that she will be able to do so. At the present stage of her illness they are likely to be upset at the prospect that her condition will worsen. At the same time, since they have a personal relationship with her, they may be even more upset if her life were not to continue. But as her condition worsens, they may become less upset at the possibility of her life ending soon.

There are also the feelings of people who do not spend much time with Mrs Green but who are involved in making decisions about her case, such as the neurologist, the ITU consultant and administrators concerned with the use of resources. They may feel sympathy for Mrs Green and for her relatives and friends, but they may also feel misgivings that the situation has arisen, since, if Mrs Green's condition had been diagnosed earlier, she would probably not have been put on the ventilator in the first place. As it is, they probably feel torn. On the one hand, they do not want to cut short Mrs Green's present situation as long as she finds it tolerable. On the other hand, they may worry that she could occupy the ventilator for many months, with no prospect that it will enable her to recover, when there may be other patients whose lives might be saved by much shorter periods on the ventilator, but for whom facilities are scarce.

In this situation the nurses may see the medical staff and managers as rather 'unfeeling' towards the patient. This is because the nurses are with the patient more than the other staff, so identify with her more strongly. They are also not aware of decisions that may have to be taken to restrict the access of other patients to the ITU. Medical and administrative staff, on the other hand, have to deal with the requirements of other patients and may have to weigh the needs of one patient against those of another.

You may have thought of other reactions that may arise in this case, but this description is enough to indicate the complexity of feelings that can be present in such a situation.

Exercise 15

If personal feelings alone are the guide, what do you think ought to be done in Mrs Green's case?

Try to answer this question before reading on.

Exercise 16

When you did Exercise 15:

1. Did you think that Mrs Green's feelings would be more important if she knew her prognosis than if she did not?
2. Did you think that Mrs Green's feelings mattered far more than anyone else's and should be met as far as possible?
3. Did you think it important to try to take into account the feelings of everyone involved?

   Answer these questions before reading on.

Exercise 17

After doing Exercises 15 and 16, do you think that feelings alone can decide what ought to be done?

It is difficult to answer 'yes' to the question in Exercise 17 because we cannot use feelings as a basis for deciding what to do until we have first answered some moral questions, such as:

1. Ought *Mrs Green's* feelings take priority over everyone else's?
2. Ought *Mr Green's* feelings take priority over everyone else's?
3. Ought Mrs Green be encouraged to know about her prognosis, so that her feelings about the actual situation can be taken into account?
4. Ought the feelings of her husband, family, friends, nurses, doctors and other professionals involved in the case be taken into account?

Exercise 18

What are your answers to these questions?
   If you answer 'yes' to any of them, can you give reasons for doing so?

One reason why you may have answered 'yes' to questions 1 or 3 is because you think it is morally right to respect the autonomy of the patient by acting in accordance with her feelings and wishes. And you may have answered 'yes' to question 4 because you think it would be unjust to ignore the autonomy or feelings of anyone involved in the case.

Although we started out thinking about personal feelings, we have reached the point at which we need to think about moral issues. So let us consider how the moral views outlined in chapters 1–4 apply to Mrs Green's case.

MORAL VIEWS

Respecting persons

The view that respecting people's autonomy is the most important element of morality suggests that Mrs Green should be consulted about her treatment and her 'informed consent' obtained to whatever course of action is taken.

In this view, she should perhaps first be asked whether or not she wishes to know her prognosis and be involved in making decisions.

If she does, possible courses of action should be explained to her and she should be treated only in ways she agrees to. But what should be done if, when she expresses her wishes, they conflict with those of the nurses or doctors? According to the need to respect the autonomy of individuals, she ought not to be treated in ways she does not want, but what if she wants to be given treatment the staff do not wish to administer? Staff, too, are people with autonomy that should be respected. Is a patient entitled to require staff to act against their wishes? Should she not respect *their* autonomy just as they respect *hers*? The principle of respecting autonomy does not give a definite answer to these questions.

What if Mrs Green does not wish to know her prognosis? In that case any consent she gives to any treatment cannot really be fully 'informed', as she does not know enough about her situation. Her autonomy can still be respected to some extent, however, by asking her whether or not she wishes to accept treatment, before it is given. But, by not wanting to know her prognosis, she really hands over to others the responsibility for making decisions and gives up much of her autonomy. Other people can respect her as a person by going along with her wish to do this.

But there still remains the obligation to respect the wishes of the other people involved in the situation and the problem of what ought to be done if their wishes conflict. If, for example, Mrs Green has increasing discomfort, her husband, relatives and friends may want the third option to be adopted – i.e. that life-prolonging treatment be suspended and painkillers that are strong enough to ensure she has no pain administered. But the staff may feel strongly that they do not wish to do this.

So, although we can see how the principle of respecting autonomy can be applied to this case, it alone does not give a sufficient guide as to how to deal with every situation that may arise.

Doing right actions and avoiding wrong ones

(the dutiful view of morality)

This is the view that actions that are wrong in themselves – actions such as deliberate killing, deliberate cruelty or acting dishonestly, unfairly or unjustly – ought to be avoided. Someone who holds this view strongly will think that such actions should not be carried out *whatever the wishes of the people involved*.

There are several ways in which the view may be applied to Mrs Green's situation.

Consider first the need to avoid acts of 'deliberate killing'.

Exercise 19

Do you think that any of the three options involves an act of 'deliberate killing'?

Some people may see taking Mrs Green off the ventilator in the third option, or withholding antibiotics in the second option, as cases of 'deliberate killing', for they may see them as acts that are carried out quite deliberately, and as likely to lead to her death.

Others would say that they are not acts of 'deliberate killing' because, if Mrs Green died:

1. the staff did not *deliberately* bring about her death; and
2. she would not have been *killed* by them.

How do they justify these claims?

They would justify the first claim by putting forward a view known as the 'doctrine of double effect'. According to this doctrine, if someone carries out an action that he knows is likely to lead to the death of another, it is only an act of deliberate killing if the person's *deliberate intention* is to kill the other person. But in this case the intention of staff in withholding antibiotics from Mrs Green, or in removing her from the ventilator, is not to kill her but to reduce the amount of suffering she will endure. We can tell that this is their intention because, if it were possible to reduce her suffering without her dying, they would have achieved their intention. They would not have to kill her by other means to achieve what they intend to do. So, according to this doctrine, the second and third options could not be seen as deliberately killing Mrs Green.

To support their claim that Mrs Green would not have been *killed* by the staff, they argue that there is an important moral difference between killing someone and letting someone die. You only kill someone if your action is the direct cause of their death, whereas you let someone die if you do not prevent other causes killing him. Taking Mrs Green off the ventilator or withholding antibiotics would not have killed her – her death would be the result of the natural causes of her illness – so the actions of staff could not be seen as acts of killing at all.

From these considerations we see that, even if people agree that deliberately killing someone is always a wrong action that ought not to be done, they may not agree on which actions are 'deliberate killing'.

Exercise 20

Do you think any of the options of treating Mrs Green involve 'deliberate cruelty'?

Some people may see the first and second options as acts of 'deliberate cruelty', since they involve deliberate actions that lead to a longer period of suffering for the patient than would allowing her to die naturally.

Against this, the argument of the 'doctrine of double effect' could again be used. This time it could be said that these options are not cases of 'deliberate cruelty', since it is not the deliberate intention of the staff to cause Mrs Green increased suffering, but rather to prolong her life, for, if they could give her a longer life without her suffering any further they would have done so. Since they would not have to make her suffer for longer to achieve their intention, the longer suffering is clearly not part of their deliberate intention.

Exercise 21

Do you find the 'doctrine of double effect' argument: more
convincing/less convincing/equally convincing when it is used to
defend staff against accusations of:

1. 'deliberate killing' or
2. 'deliberate cruelty'?

If you find the argument more convincing in one case than the
other, why is that?

By looking at these claims we see that, in the case of both 'deliberate
killing' and 'deliberate cruelty', even if people agree that these acts
should be avoided, they may not always agree which courses of action
are examples of such acts.

What of the other types of action that are considered wrong in
themselves, such as dishonest and unjust acts?

People concerned that dishonest acts should never be done will
think that if Mrs Green, her husband, relatives, friends or nurses ask
about her prognosis, they should either be told the truth or told
nothing. In this view it is morally more important to avoid dishonesty
than to avoid causing unhappiness or harm.

Those concerned to avoid injustice will regard it as unjust to ignore
the feelings and moral views of anyone involved in the case, such as
Mrs Green's relatives or friends, the nurses, doctors and resource
managers. We shall look in the next two sections at the problems of
finding out the feelings and moral views of people involved in the case
and of comparing their feelings and finding a course of action
acceptable to everyone. Those who think it important to avoid
injustice may accept that this is a problem but will think that
everyone's views should be taken into account *as far as possible* before
decisions are made.

These, then, are some of the ways in which the view that morality is a
matter of 'doing right actions and avoiding wrong ones' may apply to
this case. As with the view that morality requires us to 'respect the
autonomy of persons', it does not seem to give a definite or complete
guide as to what ought to be done.

Seeking the best consequences

(the 'useful' or utilitarian view of morality)

In this view our moral obligation is to strive to achieve the best consequences we can. This is done by assessing the likely benefits and harm to every person affected by each possible course of action. When making this assessment we should regard every person as equally important (regardless of age, sex, race, religion, etc.). If the effect on one person is likely to be greater than the effect on another, we should regard the greater effect as more important. We should then choose to act in whatever way we think will bring about the greatest amount of benefit, compatible with the least amount of harm, to all affected.

People who hold this view have different notions of 'benefit' and 'harm', but in general 'benefit' is used to mean one or more of 'pleasure', 'happiness', 'relief of suffering', 'improvement of future quality of life' and 'meeting people's needs, wishes or preferences'. By 'harm' is meant one or more of 'pain', 'misery', 'suffering', 'reduction in quality of life' and 'failing to meet people's needs, wishes or preferences'.

Exercise 22

Adopting the utilitarian approach, jot down what you see as the likely harmful and beneficial effects of the three optional courses of action in Mrs Green's case.

Below is an assessment of the likely effects of the three ways of managing Mrs Green. You may have thought of different ones, and you may not agree that some of the consequences suggested below *are* likely.

First option – harmful effects
The first option is likely to result in Mrs Green suffering for the longest amount of time, her faculties becoming worse and her pain generally increasing over a period of 18 months or so. Throughout this time the situation would be likely to cause increasing distress to her husband, family, friends, nurses and doctors as they observe her discomfort and have no hope for her recovery. After Mrs Green's death they might feel distressed that she had lived so long in pain.

In addition to the misery of Mrs Green's situation, there is the likely effect on others of her continuing to occupy the ITU bed for a long period. This could prevent its use by others for whom it might be a life-saver, enabling them to have many years of life of good quality, which would not only benefit the patients themselves but also their families and friends. The doctors, nurses and managers might also find it less distressing to work with other patients as they might feel their skills and resources were bringing greater benefits to them than to Mrs Green.

First option – beneficial effects

Against these harmful effects must be weighed the beneficial ones. At present Mrs Green is alert, thinking clearly and continuing her relationships with her husband, family, friends and nurses. The first treatment option is the one likely to prolong this state of affairs as long as possible. If it were adopted, her relations and friends could not in the future feel any distress that her ability to communicate with them had ended sooner than it might have done. Her husband, family, friends, nurses and doctors could not feel any guilt at having done anything that shortened her life.

Second option – harmful effects

The second option would be likely to give less time than the first for Mrs Green to continue her relationships with her family, friends and nurses.

It might also cause some distress and guilt among family, friends, nurses and doctors that everything had not been done to keep her alive as long as possible.

Second option – beneficial effects

The second option would result in a shorter time than the first in which the painful and distressing effects on everyone of keeping Mrs Green alive would continue.

It would also increase the likely benefits on others of earlier availability of the ITU facilities.

Third option – harmful effects

The third option would be most likely to reduce dramatically the time in which Mrs Green would remain alert and able to relate to her husband, family and friends.

After her death this option could cause more distress and guilt among family, friends, nurses and doctors that her life had not been prolonged than would either of the other two options.

Third option – beneficial effects

This option would be likely to cause the least amount of pain and suffering to Mrs Green and the least distress to her husband, family, friends, nurses and doctors at seeing her suffering.

It would also make the ITU bed and the skills of the nurses and doctors most quickly available for the benefit of other patients.

Exercise 23

You have now thought of your own ideas of the likely consequences and also read those suggested above. Basing your decision on the likely consequences alone, can you now decide what ought to be done? (Remember, when making your decision you should regard every person as equally important – regardless of age, sex, race, religion, etc. But if the effect on one person is likely to be greater than the effect on another, you should regard the greater effect as more important.)

Even taking into account the points you were asked to remember you may have found it difficult to:

1. assess the impact of different effects on different people;
2. 'weigh' the importance of various beneficial effects against various harmful ones;
3. compare the likely consequences of the three options.

You may also have found it unsatisfactory to decide on the basis of what you think is *likely* to happen, since you may feel very uncertain about the accuracy of your assessment.

Utilitarians accept that these are real difficulties with their view. But they see this as the only way to assess likely consequences. For them it is morally wrong to begin a course of action unless one honestly thinks at the time that it is likely to bring about better consequences than any other. Utilitarians consider that, as long as we carry out this assessment as well as we can with the information we have, and as long as we are sincere in our concern to produce what we see as the best likely consequences, we have acted in the morally right way. In Mrs Green's case, having carried out our assessment as members of the care team, we should take whichever option seems at the time most likely to bring about the best consequences.

So we see that, although utilitarianism gives us a method by which to make our moral judgments, it is left to us to reach our own conclusion by this method, which may not be easy.

You may want to take a break here.

Acting in accord with nature

Let us now consider how the 'nature' view applies to Mrs Green's case. As we saw in Part 1, 'nature' may be taken to mean the 'whole system of nature' or 'human nature'.

Nature as a whole
The claim that all treatments that interfere with nature are to be avoided is not one likely to be seriously maintained. For, as Exercise 9 showed, almost all treatments are attempts to stop natural processes developing in ways in which we do not want them to. So, unless someone opposes virtually all forms of medical treatment, he cannot claim that *all* interference with nature is wrong.

However some people who do not condemn all interference with nature think that there are limits to how far we should go. The problem is to define the limits of 'acceptable' interference. For example, ventilators and other components of life-support systems may be much less challenging to nature, both organically and biologically, than is a commonplace series of injections. Yet some people who oppose the use of life-support systems, because they interfere with nature too much, consider injections to be an acceptable use of medical knowledge and skills.

Some people who accept that it is difficult to define limits think that, even so, there are occasions when we can look at a range of possible treatments and generally agree that some interfere less than others with nature. These people think that on these occasions we should choose whichever treatment interferes the *least*.

Exercise 24

(Remember, in this exercise by 'nature' we mean 'nature as a whole'.)

In Mrs Green's case, which of the three treatment options do you think interferes with nature most and least?

Is there any course of action that you think interferes less than any of these options?

The first treatment option obviously interferes the most. It uses the greatest amount of interventive medicine for the longest amount of time to keep Mrs Green alive, so works hardest and longest to prevent 'nature taking its course'. The second option resists natural processes less than the first, and the third interferes least of all. So, on this basis the third option would be the preferred one.

However, there is a further course of action that most people would agree would interfere with nature even less than the third option: if Mrs Green were simply taken off the ventilator and not given any treatment to make her comfortable, she would experience the pain someone would *naturally* feel in her medical condition. So according to the principle of 'interfering with nature the least', this is the action we should choose.

But even the most ardent supporter of minimum interference is unlikely to agree to this course of action. Why is this? Probably because when someone says, 'We should do whatever interferes with nature the least', he means 'we should interfere with nature the least amount *that is necessary to achieve our aims*'.

But this leaves us with the question 'What ought our aims to be?' Ought we aim to keep Mrs Green alive for as long as possible, or to make her suffering as brief as possible? In other words, we are back with our original moral problem, and the principle that we should interfere with nature as little as possible has not solved it.

From these considerations we see that, if by 'nature' we mean 'nature as a whole':

1. it is difficult to define limits of acceptable levels of interference with nature;
2. the principle that we should 'interfere with nature as little as possible' amounts to saying either that we should give virtually no medical treatment or that we must first decide the aim of our treatment on some other moral grounds.

Let us now think of nature as 'human nature'.

Human nature
Now try Exercise 25.

Exercise 25

Which of the three options do you think is most in accord with human nature?

You may have found it difficult to reach a clear answer to this question because 'human nature' can include so many factors.

It is, for example, natural for humans to use their intelligence to strive for whatever gives them emotional satisfaction, and since Mrs Green is alert and loved, it is natural to strive to keep her alive as long as possible, as in the first option. But the desire to avoid prolonging pain and suffering is also natural to human beings; so, to use human skills to enable Mrs Green to die as painlessly as possible after the least amount of suffering, as in the third option, is also in accord with human nature. And as the second option strives to keep Mrs Green alive for some time, but then does not prolong her suffering once it becomes worse, it can be seen to be in accord with both 'natural' impulses. So it is not easy to choose between the three options by deciding that one of them is most in accord with 'human nature'.

In fact in this situation deciding what we ought to do by appealing to 'human nature' would, of course, be much more complicated than we have suggested so far. Those involved in Mrs Green's case would have a variety of feelings and emotions – far more than just the two impulses we have selected. All of these feelings would occur quite 'naturally', even though some may be regarded as 'bad'. For instance, some people may long for Mrs Green to die quickly so they are free of their anxiety about her. As it is natural to have such feelings, they must be taken into account if we are concerned to act in accord with whatever feelings are part of human nature.

Since there may be a variety of feelings in favour of different courses of action, it may seem most 'natural' to act in accordance with whichever feelings are thought to be most dominant at the time. But it may be difficult to judge which ones *are* dominant. To make a decision on this basis one person – or a group of people – would have to be very well informed about the strength of feelings of everyone involved, and measure the strength of their feelings against each other. This would need everyone to co-operate by expressing their reactions as openly as possible, and would not be achieved easily.

In addition, the feelings that are dominant are likely to change. As long as Mrs Green remains alert and 'able to cope', dominant feelings may seem to be in favour of keeping her alive. At this point the first option ought to be followed. But once Mrs Green begins to suffer more, the desire to let her suffering come to an end may seem strongest, so the second option should be followed. Later the desire to avoid further suffering as much as possible may seem so strong that the third option should be adopted.

A further problem is that making a decision in this way could require discussion of many of the moral issues that people who appeal to 'human nature' often hope to avoid. For once we start comparing and measuring people's feelings, we have to consider whether the feelings of some people – e.g. Mrs Green and her husband – should be given more importance than the feelings of others. So, before we can decide how to apply an assessment of people's 'natural' feelings, we find we have to think about *other* moral issues.

From these considerations we see that any attempt to judge which courses of action are most 'in accordance with human nature' requires far more complex considerations than a simple judgment about what people 'naturally feel' in a particular situation.

Doing God's will

As we saw in Part 1, religious traditions vary in the way they interpret God's will. Although all traditions agree that we have a general obligation to prevent ill health, care for the sick and preserve life, and that it is normally wrong to kill a person deliberately, religions vary in the way they interpret these general obligations and in the way they apply them to particular situations. To look at all the ways in which they may be applied to Mrs Green's situation would require detailed consideration far beyond the scope of this book. Consequently, all we can do here is indicate how some of the views of the main religious traditions may relate to her case.

As far as the need to avoid 'deliberate killing' is concerned, many Roman Catholics adopt the 'doctrine of double effect' and also hold the view that there is an important moral difference between *killing* and *letting die* (see p. 48), so they would regard the second and third options as permissible. Some Catholics, however, while seeing these options as permissible, would regard the preservation of human life as the most important duty, so would consider the first option as better than the other two. Others might be torn between the value of preserving Mrs Green's life and the value of reducing her suffering.

Many Protestants might be equally torn, for many would emphasise the moral importance of 'duty to each other'. In health care this is usually taken to mean that the most important duty of carers is to their patient, for example, to put the patient's interests before any other consideration, or to regard the patient's wishes as more important than those of anyone else. But in Mrs Green's case it may not be clear what *is* in her interest. Is it more in her interest for her to be kept alive as long as possible or to suffer as little as possible? Some Protestants might resolve this dilemma by combining the idea of 'duty to the patient's interest' with the more general Christian ideal of 'being loving', which is often seen as concern to reduce suffering. On this basis they might see it as in her interest for her to suffer as little as possible, so might choose the third option.

Other Protestants, however, might interpret 'being loving' as a concern to minimise the suffering of *everyone*. Applied to Mrs Green's case, this would require an assessment of how each option would affect everyone in the situation, not just the patient, and would lead to an approach similar to the utilitarian method already discussed above. But loving concern for everyone could conflict with concern for the patient's best interests, since the least suffering for everyone might be achieved by one option, whereas Mrs Green's best interests might be served by another.

Some religions lay greater stress than others on the need to preserve life. In Judaism, for instance, sick or injured people are generally seen as having a duty to seek life-saving treatment, and health-care workers as having a duty to preserve life by whatever means are medically possible – no practices are considered unacceptable on the grounds that they are 'unnatural'. Some Jews see the preservation of life as so important that the wishes of patients who refuse life-saving or life-prolonging treatment may be ignored. Because of this great importance in Judaism of preserving life, it is normally considered wrong to withdraw treatment from a terminally ill patient as long as life can be maintained. Many Jews might, therefore, regard the first option as right. However, for some it is permissible in a terminal case not to delay a death that is very close, so they might think the second or third options should be considered once Mrs Green's death becomes imminent.

In Hinduism it is generally important to prevent suffering, but even more important to avoid violation of life, so it would usually be thought wrong to take a person's life in order to relieve his suffering. As long as they did not see the third option as any form of 'deliberate killing', many Hindus would probably prefer this option, since it is the one likely to prevent most suffering. The other two options might also be rejected by many Hindus on the grounds that they see them as interventions to prevent a death that would otherwise be imminent.

Many Muslims, too, might be against efforts to prolong life or to hasten death, if they see them as attempts to interfere with the will of God. Muslims who take this view might think that treatment should be carried out as long as it is concerned to improve poor health or relieve suffering, but not if its only purpose is to delay death. So they might find the first option acceptable as long as it cures infections and relieves suffering but, once there is no prospect of improving Mrs Green's condition or relieving her suffering, they might consider that there should be no further intervention, and the third option should be adopted.

These brief glances are not attempts to explain the views of any of the major religious traditions. They are merely indications of the way in which *some* aspects of thought in each of the traditions may relate to this particular case. Within a religious tradition there may be several perspectives, and we have not been able to consider any of them properly here.

REVIEW

Having applied the most commonly-held general moral views to Mrs Green's case, we see that none of them gives an immediate, cut-and-dried answer as to what is right in this particular situation.

This is not really surprising, since for most of us making a moral decision is frequently a matter of trying to work out how best to apply our *general* moral views to a *particular* set of circumstances, and there is often room for interpretation of how this should be done.

Individuals in any group of health-care workers are likely to have different opinions on which of the moral views we have considered are the most important. I hope this short book has helped you to understand how each of the views can be seen as important for morality, and so helped you to appreciate the sincerity of people who hold them. If you can understand how people with various views see their opinions as *justified and reasonable*, you are in a good position to discuss moral problems with them and to look for courses of action that are morally acceptable to all concerned.

Unfortunately, you may often be working in a situation in which all decisions are made by others and little or no attention is paid to what you think. This book should help you to understand the considerations by which other people reach their decisions. And, if you find you disagree with a decision about the management of a patient, you may at least be able to appreciate the reasons for the decision. This may make you happier about caring for a patient in a way you would not have chosen. Of course, you may see that the reasons for the decision are not moral ones at all, in which case, you will form your own ideas about the people you are working with.

6 Further cases to consider

Here are more cases for you to consider:

1. Jane is a young woman who is dying fairly comfortably in a hospice. She is being administered diamorphine via a pump. Relatives and friends visit her constantly and the nurses realise that the pump has been tampered with to increase the dosage. They talk to her visitors and make it clear that they know what has happened. It is obvious that Jane, her family and friends are all convinced that it is right that they should do all they can to ensure she has as painless a death as possible. Although they promise not to interfere with the pump again, they continue to do so. What action should the nurses take?

2. A psychiatric nurse develops a relationship of trust with a patient who tells her in confidence that she was sexually abused as a child. The nurse considers this fact to be very relevant to the patient's illness. Should the nurse write the information in the patient's 'care plan'?

3. A nurse on an acute medical ward frequently has to decide when patients should be discharged and, when doing so, feels under considerable pressure. On the one hand, she is constantly told to discharge patients as soon as possible. On the other, she thinks that she sometimes sends elderly patients home too early in their recovery from strokes or broken bones. What factors should she bear in mind when making these decisions? Should she consider refusing to discharge patients?

4. A nurse has been asked by the relatives of a patient not to tell him that his illness is terminal, as they think he would be very upset if he knew his situation. After she has cared for him for some time on night duty, he asks her whether he is dying. He says he wants

to know the truth as he wants to prepare himself and his relations for his death. The nurse is convinced he is strong enough to be told about his condition. What should she do?

Exercise 26

1. What do you think people who hold the various moral views we have looked at may say about these cases? To remind you, here is a list of the moral views:

   - Respecting personal autonomy.
   - The 'dutiful' view (doing right actions/avoiding wrong actions).
   - The utilitarian view (seeking the best consequences).
   - A combination of the dutiful and utilitarian views.
   - Acting in accord with 'nature as a whole' or 'human nature'.
   - Doing God's will.

2. The Codes of Conduct (pp. 65–67) reflect many of the moral views we have considered. Look at the Codes and consider how much guidance they give for dealing with these cases.

7 | Checklist of questions

The following questions express the moral concerns of the views we have considered.

You will find this a useful checklist if ever you are faced with a difficult decision and want to think about all possible moral aspects. You will also find it a useful means of anticipating the moral questions that people may raise about a situation. (You may not think all the questions are relevant to a particular situation.)

1. How much should the patient be – told?
                                   – consulted?
2. How much should the relatives and friends be – told?
                                              – consulted?
3. How much should various members of the caring team be
   – told?
   – consulted?
4. Should informed consent be obtained for treatment?
5. Are anyone's rights being infringed?
6. Are there courses of action that may be seen as right or wrong 'in themselves'?
7. Is there any deliberate intention to curtail life?
8. Is 'sanctity of life' an overriding principle in this case?
9. What counts as 'harm' in this case?
10. Is there any deliberate intention to cause unnecessary 'harm'?
11. Are the needs, views and feelings of everyone involved being given just and fair consideration?
12. Are resources being made available on a fair basis?
13. How can benefits be maximised?
14. How can suffering be minimised?
15. What is the most beneficial use of resources?
16. Are there any courses of action that may be seen as 'unnatural'?

17. Are there any religious perspectives of the patient, relatives, friends and members of the caring team that should be considered?
18. How do any of the above considerations affect the professional duties of the carers – to the patient?
                                              – to each other?
19. What *other* questions are relevant to the case before you?

Exercise 27

Can you identify the moral views from which these questions come?

---

8 Codes of conduct

UKCC CODE OF PROFESSIONAL CONDUCT FOR THE NURSE, MIDWIFE AND HEALTH VISITOR

(Reprinted by kind permission of the UKCC.)

Each registered nurse, midwife and health visitor shall act, at all times, in such a manner as to justify public trust and confidence, to uphold and enhance the good standing and reputation of the profession, to serve the interests of society, and above all to safeguard the interests of individual patients and clients.

Each registered nurse, midwife and health visitor is accountable for his or her practice, and, in the exercise of professional accountability shall:

1. Act always in such a way as to promote and safeguard the well being and interests of patients/clients.
2. Ensure that no action or omission on his/her part or within his/her sphere of influence is detrimental to the condition or safety of patients/clients.
3. Take every reasonable opportunity to maintain and improve professional knowledge and competence.
4. Acknowledge any limitations of competence and refuse in such cases to accept delegated functions without first having received instruction in regard to those functions and having been assessed as competent.
5. Work in a collaborative and co-operative manner with other health care professionals and recognise and respect their particular contributions within the health care team.
6. Take account of the customs, values and spiritual beliefs of patients/clients.
7. Make known to an appropriate person or authority any conscientious objection which may be relevant to professional practice.

8. Avoid any abuse of the privileged relationship which exists with patients/clients and of the privileged access allowed to their property, residence or workplace.

9. Respect confidential information obtained in the course of professional practice and refrain from disclosing such information without the consent of the patient/client, or a person entitled to act on his/her behalf, except where disclosure is required by law or by the order of a court or is necessary in the public interest.

10. Have regard to the environment of care and its physical, psychological and social effects on patients/clients, and also to the adequacy of resources, and make known to appropriate persons or authorities any circumstances which could place patients/clients in jeopardy or which militate against safe standards of practice.

11. Have regard to the workload of and the pressures on professional colleagues and subordinates and take appropriate action if these are seen to be such as to constitute abuse of the individual practitioner and/or to jeopardise safe standards of practice.

12. In the context of the individual's own knowledge, experience and sphere of authority assist peers and subordinates to develop professional competence in accordance with their needs.

13. Refuse to accept any gift, favour or hospitality which might be interpreted as seeking to exert undue influence to obtain preferential consideration.

14. Avoid the use of professional qualifications in the promotion of commercial products in order not to compromise the independence of professional judgment on which patients/clients rely.

Notice to all Registered Nurses, Midwives and Health Visitors
This Code of Professional Conduct is issued by the United Kingdom Central Council for Nursing, Midwifery and Health Visiting.

It is issued for the guidance and advice of all registered nurses, midwives and health visitors.

Further explanatory notes, discussion papers or comments on specific points in the Code of Professional Conduct may be issued by the Council from time to time.

The Code will be subject to periodic review by the Council.

The Council expects members of the profession to recognise it as their responsibility (as well as the Council's) to re-appraise the relevance of the Code to the professional and social context in which they practise.

The Council will welcome suggestions and comments for consideration in its periodic review of the Code of Professional Conduct. Such suggestions and comments should be sent to:

**United Kingdom
Central Council
for Nursing,
Midwifery and
Health Visiting**
(PC Division)
23 Portland Place
London W1N 3AF

RCN CODE OF PROFESSIONAL CONDUCT DISCUSSION DOCUMENT

This discussion document was produced by the Royal College of Nursing in the 1970s as a contribution to the debate on moral values in nursing practice. Out of this debate came the UKCC Code of Professional Conduct. Although the UKCC Code supercedes this discussion document, it is valuable to read the document as it discusses many of the concerns that led to the formulation of the current UKCC Code.

(Reprinted by kind permission of the Royal College of Nursing.)

Text

I Introduction

The profession of nursing has a commitment which is shared with other health care professions to promote optimal standards of health, combat disease and disability and alleviate suffering. A code of professional conduct is required in order to make explicit those moral standards which should guide professional decisions in these matters, and in order to encourage responsible moral decision making throughout the profession. It is recognised that no code can do justice to every individual case and therefore that any set of principles must remain constantly open to discussion both within the nursing profession and outside it.

Discussion

1 The starting point of this code is the recognition that nursing is now a profession in its own right, with all the responsibility which that entails. It shares with other professions – notably medicine and social work – the goal of improving the health prospects of all members of that society which grants it the right to practise. Because ideas about health goals vary from individual to individual, and because nurses have considerable influence (and on occasion power) over patients or clients whose needs and handicap often render them especially vulnerable, a code of conduct is needed to provide guidelines for professional practice. Such a code ought to be continuously developed and refined by sustained discussion among nurses themselves, and by consultation between nurses and those who can speak for other professions and for the general public.

Codes are never a substitute for personal moral integrity, and they can often be hardened into legal formulae. It must therefore be stressed that the purpose of this code is not to devise grounds for disciplinary proceedings (or any similar purpose), but rather to provide a clear and comprehensive document for further discussion, particularly during periods of professional training.

II Responsibility to patients or clients

The primary responsibility of nurses is to protect and enhance the wellbeing and dignity of each individual person in their care. As members of professional teams nurses should recognise and accept responsibility for the total effect of nursing and medical care on individuals. This responsibility is in no way affected by the type of origin of the person's need or illness or by his age, sex, mental status, social class, ethnic origins, nationality or personal beliefs. Therefore it follows that:

1. Nursing care should be directed towards the preservation, or restoration, as far as is possible, of a person's ability to function normally and independently within his own chosen environment.

1. As a form of social occupation nursing serves several ends: it provides paid employment to a large section of society; it gives individuals a sense of intellectual achievement and job satisfaction; and it offers congenial and rewarding inter- and intra-professional relationships. But none of these should take precedence over the *primary* end of nursing, which is to enable people to live their own lives as fully and freely as possible by providing professional counsel and care according to particular needs.

2. Discrimination against particular individuals, for whatever reason, should never be tolerated.

2. Entering the nursing profession involves a commitment to the service of persons, each of whom merits individual respect. At times nurses may have prejudices against patients or clients because they consider that they are largely responsible for their own misfortune or because they cannot feel any sympathy for their particular form of distress. But the adoption of a professional attitude requires that all those who need nursing care should receive it without discrimination. No group of patients or clients should be regarded as unworthy or undeserving of professional concern.

3. During episodes of illness the autonomy of patients should be maintained throughout treatment, restrictions being imposed only when these are demonstrably necessary for their own wellbeing, or for the safety of others; and the active participation of patients in their own treatment should be facilitated by means of open and sensitive communication.

3. Nurses share in responsibility for the effect of the multi-disciplinary treatment methods of modern medicine on personal health and freedom. In particular, the routines of hospitals and health institutions and other organisational structures may unnecessarily remove the dignity and independence of patients, thereby diminishing their overall health prospects. In view of this a fundamental aspect of the nurse's responsibility to the patient can be seen as the maintenance and restoration of personal autonomy. This is principally achieved by skilled nursing care of each individual, with an understanding of the context of his illness or disability and with careful attention being paid to communication with him, especially during periods of anxiety. In this context it should be noted that the best source of information about the patient is usually the patient himself and that regular and relaxed discussions with relatives can increase the nurse's understanding of the patient's circumstances and of possible ways in which he can be helped to achieve an optimal level of living. It is recognised that dealing with violent or potentially violent patients raises particularly difficult problems in relation to restraint and patients' freedom. It is essential that clear guidelines are given to all those who have such patients in their care to ensure that prejudice and mutual fear between patients and staff do not worsen the situation. (See the guidelines offered by the DHSS on the basis of joint advice from the Rcn and the Royal College of Psychiatrists. *The Management of Violent or Potentially Violent Hospital Patients* HC(76)11).

4. Measures which jeopardise the safety of patients, such as unnecessary treatments, hazardous experimental procedures and the withdrawal of professional services during employment disputes, should be actively opposed by the profession as a whole.

4. Actions which betray people's confidence in the professional integrity of nurses diminish the ability of the profession to be of help. For this reason the nursing profession should be clearly seen to be opposed to exploitation of vulnerability, for example: Treatment and Experimentation – inappropriate treatment, risky experimentation or experimentation without proper consent; or Industrial Action – the removal of professional services which puts patients at risk.

Although choice of treatments and the initiation of clinical research projects is usually solely a medical responsibility, nurses have the right and the duty to express opinions about the effect of such procedures on the patients under their care. (For instance a nurse may question whether the dignity of a dying patient is being respected by procedures employed to delay death; and the design of an experiment involving discomfort or risk to patients may be questioned by nurses asked to co-operate in the experiment.)

Nurses are entitled to equitable wages and conditions of employment and should be free to enter into appropriate negotiations with their employers. But since seriously ill people are in no position to protect themselves when professional aid is withdrawn, disruption of services by strike action and threats to do so contravene the nurse's commitment to service of patients and should be publicly opposed, whether the action is carried out by nurses or by other professions and occupations involved in health care.

5. Information about patients or clients should be treated with the utmost confidence and respect, and should not be divulged to persons outwith the primary care or treatment team without the person's consent, except in exceptional circumstances.

5. In unusual circumstances it may be necessary to disclose confidential information for the well-being of the patient or others in the nurse's care, but this should never be done without full consultation with relatives and with medical and nursing colleagues, and whenever possible the patient should be told why such a disclosure was felt to be necessary.

III Responsibility for professional standards

The professional authority of nurses is based upon their training and experience in day to day care of ill persons at home or in hospital; and in the enhancement of positive health in the community at large. All members of the nursing profession have a responsibility to continue to develop their knowledge and skill in these matters.

III This claim to professional status implies that nurses have particular forms of knowledge and skill in health care which are not shared by other professions and which thereby give them the authority to institute nursing procedures and make decisions and recommendations about correct nursing care.

This claim must be substantiated by the profession as a whole through the establishment of training procedures and the maintenance of competence at all levels within the profession and by continued research into new and improved methods of nursing care.

Individual nurses have the responsibility to be self-critical of their professional performance and to seek to adapt it to changing needs and new techniques of care.

IV Responsibility to colleagues

In general, relationships with colleagues in nursing and in other health care professions should be determined according to what will maximise the benefit of those in their care.

IV The goal of 'whole person treatment' determines how nurses should relate professionally to their fellow nurses and to members of other health care professions. It is assumed that the more there is co-operation and communication between the different people caring for the patient, the more the patient's needs are likely to be understood and catered for. (As noted in the previous section, the patient himself has also a great deal to contribute to such full understanding, as do his relatives.)

1. Professional relationships between nurses should be regulated according to the level of knowledge, experience and skill of each nurse. Clear chains of command should be established to deal with emergency situations, but except in such situations, free discussion of the reasons for established procedures should be encouraged at all levels.

1. The nursing 'hierarchy' can be seen to be necessary to ensure that decisions are taken by those who should have the requisite knowledge and experience, but on the other hand junior members of staff can often bring fresh insights about patients or be more successful in gaining the patient's confidence. For this reason an atmosphere of friendly questioning and discussion between staff at different levels can improve the quality of care as well as making nurse education more effective. (Obviously clear lines of authority are needed for situations in which rapid decisions have to be made.)

2. Professional relationships between nurses and doctors should be regulated according to the particular expertise of each profession. In the case of medical treatments nurses are under an obligation to carry out a doctor's instructions except where they have a good reason to believe that harm will be caused to the patient by so doing. In cases in which nurses' continuous contact with the patient has given them a different insight into the patient's medical needs, they are under moral obligation to communicate this to the doctor in charge of the case. Nurses should support the multi-disciplinary case-conference approach to treatment decisions, and should improve their ability to participate actively in such conferences.

2. Nurses are not trained to diagnose illness or to prescribe medical treatment. They must therefore normally carry out doctors' instructions in these matters and help maintain the patient's confidence in his medical advisors. But nurses are in a unique position to observe the condition of the patient at all hours of day and night and have received basic instruction in drug dosages, effects of treatment, etc. For this reason they are morally obliged to question medical instructions which they believe will cause the patient harm or unnecessary distress (see Section II) even though they may fear adverse effects on their career from doing so. Ideally, however, this should not entail a confrontation between doctor and nurse, but should arise naturally in the context of ongoing inter-professional discussions in case conferences. Part of the professional training of nurses should prepare them to take part in such conferences from their own professional standpoint.

3. Professional relationships between nurses and members of other health care professions should be based upon respect for each other's area of expertise and on the desire to gain a fuller understanding of the patient's or client's needs. Procedures should be established for regular inter-professional consultations.

3. In the case of other professions which may have contact with patients or clients (e.g. para-medical professions, social workers, hospital chaplains and other clergy) nurses should be concerned to establish relationships of trust. This should promote a mutual understanding of professional roles enabling the patient/client to derive maximum benefit from the work of the caring team.

V Professional responsibility and personal responsibility

As citizens of a state and as private individuals nurses should defend and actively pursue those moral values to which their profession is committed, namely, individual autonomy, parity of treatment and the pursuit of health. In some circumstances this may require protest against, and opposition to, social and political conditions which are detrimental to human wellbeing; and in others, the altering of personal habits which set a poor example in health care. In all other respects nurses have the right to regulate their private lives according to their own standards of morality, provided their style of life does not cast doubts on the integrity and trustworthiness of their profession.

V Because nursing finds its origins partly in religious orders, there may be unrealistic expectations both within the profession and among the general public about the degree of personal dedication to which modern nurses should aspire. Like other professionals, nurses have the right to conduct their private lives without undue interference from colleagues or employers. Also like other professionals, however, the choice of a personal service career commits the nurse to certain moral views. Nurses cannot strive to alleviate disease and suffering without becoming aware of the social circumstances which bring it about or which inhibit the provision of effective remedies. It follows that nurses should be concerned with political and social issues, whenever these are relevant to the prevention of disease or the delivery of health care. Similarly in the sphere of personal conduct, nurses should strive to 'practise what they preach' to avoid personal habits which are known to be detrimental to health. (For example, doctors and nurses are particularly at risk for drug and alcohol addiction – a factor which seems to demand closer supportive attention from their respective professions.)

In addition to setting a good example in healthy styles of life, nurses need to inspire confidence in patients in order to be able to help them fully. This does not imply 'angelic' purity of life – merely the following of standards of honesty and of moral seriousness which would be expected from any member of society who has responsibility for the welfare of others.

INTERNATIONAL COUNCIL OF NURSES CODE FOR NURSES

(Reprinted by kind permission of the International Council of Nurses.)

The fundamental responsibility of the nurse is fourfold: to promote health, to prevent illness, to restore health and to alleviate suffering.

The need for nursing is universal. Inherent in nursing is respect for life, dignity and rights of man. It is unrestricted by considerations of nationality, race, creed, colour, age, sex, politics or social status.

Nurses render health services to the individual, the family and the community and coordinate their services with those of related groups.

Nurses and people

The nurse's primary responsibility is to those people who require nursing care.

The nurse, in providing care, promotes an environment in which the values, customs and spiritual beliefs of the individual are respected.

The nurse holds in confidence personal information and uses judgment in sharing this information.

Nurses and practice

The nurse carries personal responsibility for nursing practice and for maintaining competence by continual learning.

The nurse maintains the highest standards of nursing care possible within the reality of a specific situation.

The nurse uses judgment in relation to individual competence when accepting and delegating responsibilities.

The nurse when acting in a professional capacity should at all times maintain standards of personal conduct which reflect credit upon the profession.

Nurses and society

The nurse shares with other citizens the responsibility for initiating and supporting action to meet the health and social needs of the public.

Nurses and co-workers

The nurse sustains a cooperative relationship with co-workers in nursing and other fields.

The nurse takes appropriate action to safeguard the individual when his care is endangered by a co-worker or any other person.

Nurses and the profession

The nurse plays the major role in determining and implementing desirable standards of nursing practice and nursing education.

The nurse is active in developing a core of professional knowledge.

The nurse, acting through the professional organization, participates in establishing and maintaining equitable social and economic working conditions in nursing.

Suggestions for application by nursing educators, practitioners, administrators and nurses' associations of concepts of the Code for Nurses

The **Code for Nurses** is a guide for action based on values and needs of society. It will have meaning only if it becomes a living document applied to the realities of human behaviour in a changing society.

In order to achieve its purpose the **Code** must be understood, internalized and utilized by nurses in all aspects of their work. It must be put before and be continuously available to students and practitioners in their mother tongue, throughout their study and work lives. For practical application in the local setting, the **Code** should be studied in conjunction with information relevant to the specific situation which would guide the nurse in selecting priorities and scope for action in nursing.

These suggestions need to be adapted, expanded and supplemented by additional items.

Exercise 28

Which of the moral views that we have looked at are reflected in points in these Codes?

Further Reading

General introduction to nursing ethics

Burnard P and Chapman C M (1988) *Professional and Ethical Issues in Nursing*. Chichester: John Wiley and Sons.

Rumbold G (1986) *Ethics in Nursing Practice*. Eastbourne: Baillière Tindall.

Thompson I E, Melia K M and Boyd K M (1983) *Nursing Ethics*. London: Churchill Livingstone.

Tschudin V (1986) *Ethics in Nursing*. London: Heinemann.

Ethical theories in relation to health care

Beauchamp T L and Childress J F (1983) *Principles of Bio-Medical Ethics.* New York: Oxford University Press.

Seedhouse D (1988) *Ethics, The Heart of Health Care*. Chichester: John Wiley and Sons.

Discussions of particular ethical issues raised in this book

e.g. respect for persons, autonomy and rights, informed consent, treatment of the terminally ill, killing and letting die, doctrine of double effect.

Campbell R and Collinson D (1988) *Ending Lives*. Oxford: Blackwell.

Downie R S and Calman K C (1987) *Healthy Respects: Ethics in Healthcare*. London: Faber and Faber.

Faulder C (1985) *Whose Body Is It?* London: Virago.

Glover J (1977) *Causing Death and Saving Lives*. Harmondsworth: Pelican.

Harris J (1990) *The Value of Life*. London: Routledge and Kegan Paul.

Most of these books contain extensive bibliographies.

Index